STRENGTH IS NOT OPTIONAL

BY JEREMIAH CLARK

DISCLAIMER

I am not licensed in the areas of fitness, nutrition, or mental health. The information shared in this book is from my point of view, and from my personal opinion and experiences only.

Please consult your physician before attempting to try any of the fitness, nutrition, or mental health ideas mentioned is this book.

DEDICATION

I want to dedicate this book to all who are seeking more out of their life.
To those who seek the truth.
To those who see the truth that beauty and pain are unfortunately a necessary connection and balance in this world.
To those who choose to embrace strength and kindness together.

I truly thank you for investing your time, energy, and resources in this book.

Be Strong and Be Kind

Jeremiah Clark

ACKNOWLEDGMENTS

I want to thank my wife for being by my side all these years. She has been a vital part of my life in helping me become the man I am today, and want to be tomorrow.

To my three kids, I will always be by your side fighting for you and all you dream for in your lives. Thanks for having the patience and trust in me making decisions and choices in your life that was and still is needed as I take on life and keep punching through the tough moments while at the same time thinking what is best for the family.

I want to thank all my close friends and family. I have needed so much help in all areas of my life at one point or another. You have been there to step in and save the day. You know who you are, and I will never forget those who sacrificed their time, energy, and resources to my family and me.

I want to thank my friend, Tom Russell, for believing in me and taking a chance on a naive writer who needed a friend's guidance with a writing background.

His guidance and passion to help others has been so important in completing these two books and making them available to read.

It may be a little weird and a shock to my ego. I want to humble myself and thank even those who have created negative situations and hard choices for me to make.

I would definitely not be at this place in my life physically, mentally, or spiritually without the help of many people both past and present. There have been those who left either a positive or negative impact on me. No matter which one was left on me, I needed them both. Both types were helpful, and even vital in shaping my character.

<u>**STRENGTH IS NOT OPTIONAL**</u>

INTRODUCTION

STRENGTH IS NOT OPTIONAL

It was two years in the making. I received the email saying that my very first book was written and was online and ready to buy.

I was very excited as I went on social media to passionately tell others that the book I finally had enough courage to write and complete was ready for all to read.

I titled the book "It's All About Faith~Family~Fitness." Even though everyone has uniqueness to their life, I still wanted to share mine in the book. I shared about how our rough relationship started with teenage pregnancy and marriage. I wrote about faith, both how I rejected and embraced it. I shared how both faith and fitness shaped my life's direction on how I lived my life, lead my family, loved my wife, and the impact I wanted to leave on the world.

Sounds like I have it all figured out, right? That couldn't be further from the truth.

If anything, life is more complicated than I thought. After people read the book, it lead to others sharing their stories with me. It opened my eyes further on how much pain people are experiencing in the world physically, mentally, and spiritually.

There definitely was a pattern. Most people agreed that those areas of life were important to evaluate. Most people were still frustrated after trying to embrace faith and fitness in their life, but still struggled by the complexity of having it be a part of their lives every day.

I was frustrated and torn by many of the responses, because I could only imagine dealing with some of the pain and suffering that they were dealing with, making it hard to trust the idea that faith was connected to their personal lives, or in other cases that working out every day is too consuming and not that important on the to-do list.

Everyone deals with pain and suffering in their life. You can possibly relate to it or have similar experiences, but no two lives are the same, or the process of dealing with it. We are connected to one another in so many ways; we are not so divided as society makes us out to be.

The other frustration was they put those areas of their lives a top priority, but the true level of commitment was not there yet, even though they believed it had already been met. I wanted to push the idea that nobody is perfect, but maybe more effort and discipline was needed to truly make changes.

The year my book was published I was able to speak at a handful of different platforms such as churches, sports teams, fitness clubs, and my job used the book as part of their leadership program. I expressed my thoughts on spending effort to take on the principles I talked about, and challenged themselves in those areas so maybe the changes they were looking for in life would start appearing.

Just as I struggled with the same areas, I understood that you can't be pushed into believing something needs to be in your life until you are ready for it. I tried to remember that with each conversation I had.

A few months into that same year, as you know, life can hit harder than anyone, and our family was hit often those next few months. It's something that will be a part of everyone's life, but to put it bluntly, it sucks to deal with...death. We had four people close to us who died, and it became tough to cope with in a five-month period.

Having little experience with death, we were all struggling as a family. Finally, I researched online to see what type of advice would help me cope with the pain. Each website offered similar and helpful advice, but something that stood out to me was there was always one absolute vital core thought on each one of the sites. You must deal with the death, and never hide the emotions or withhold feelings, and withdraw from life to avoid emotional suffering.

The websites all warned that if you were to try to bundle up the emotions and not deal with them that the pain and emotions intensified, and it becomes even harder to deal with, and can eventually lead to bigger mental health issues later.

They understood the desire to avoid the pain and just move on with life, but it just doesn't work like that. You must embrace the healing process of dealing with the emotions, and over time it will become easier to deal with and hopefully not be as intense as time goes on.

From that day on, I purposely tried all their methods of dealing with the losses, and it worked as time went on. Also, from that day forward, I applied the thought of just dealing with problems head on instead of complaining about them, and letting time slip away. It just became a frequent way to deal with things that came up on any given day. I started reading more books and watching YouTube videos on how to be successful and achieving more out of life.

As I read those books, watched those videos and had conversations with others about the first book, I felt there was a certain momentum with others reading it throughout the year. But a few unfortunate and awkward situations and thoughts came center stage. I learned to now believe people's actions more than their words. I also realized that it was time to step up the intensity and discipline in anything that we want to have happen in our life. I mean everything.

I truly believe that we all have this unknown potential in our life, and the desire to be the best we can be in every area we want to be known for in our life.

We need to embrace and change our mindset of thinking that certain characteristic traits are too boring, too routine, too unattainable to have in our lives every single day.

Just like a best friend or a loved one wants only to see you succeed in your life, so does self discipline. Self discipline is your friend, not your enemy, and something you should desire to have in your life.

Don't be fooled otherwise. Just as I am learning now, and will continue to learn this, we all need to accept this now. It unfortunately doesn't matter if you or I agree with this thought or not, but discipline is the key. It's a way to accomplish all your dreams, goals, and will give you the freedom later on after applying all of this self discipline over time.

Yes, it will be tough, and it will not be fun, and may be boring at times, but the promise is there that it will change you however you want to be physically, mentally, or spiritually over time depending on your desire and discipline. What do we need to accomplish this?

Strength is the key. We need this in all areas: physically, mentally, and spiritually.

What do you think? Do you believe you have this unknown strength inside you? I believe we all do, and I'm sharing my experiences with you on this, and trying to convince you on this, because I want everyone in the world to love one another. I truly believe that if people applied this mindset, it would improve their lives and the people surrounding them.

Let's do this, because I believe that if we all have this unknown potential, then inside of us also is this unknown potential way of achieving it. So one thing is certain:

Strength is not optional.

CHAPTER ONE

A NEW KIND OF STRONG

Have you ever had a breakdown? I'm not talking about the bad ones, like chair throwing or f-bombing everyone. I'm talking about the ones that at the end of them you are so thankful and humbled to have them. They are extremely rare to have.

These are moments that are very private. You are alone, and probably tired, sad, angry, with tears streaming down your face, and you are disgusted with the status quo. At the end of the moment, usually your life has been altered in some way.

The conversation with yourself will be emotional, sincere and very real. That is the type of emotions and conversations most of the world wants to have with people. But you know how rare that is.

Why do people avoid those types of moments? Well, let me clarify, and avoid the first breakdowns I described. Those are not good on so many levels. In fact, it shows weakness, not strength.

In honor of my desire to be very transparent through this book, I need to share my emotions of a few breakdowns that helped set up a course correction each time.

I was young when one happened. It was the spring of my seventh grade year, and I had just lost my first track race. I was favored to win, because I had been the fastest kid in school for a while. When I crossed that finish line in almost last place I was devastated.

That evening, looking out my bedroom window, I was frustrated by my lack of discipline of not training during the summer like the winner of the race probably did. I had this determination, this anger in my eyes that I had never experienced before.

I felt empowered, like I now had the answers and a plan to fix this problem forever. It was one of those thoughts that popped into my head, the one where you don't know if it was from a higher power, or an idea coming from deep within your mind, or both.

"You are going to start working out, and it will be a big part of your life," I resolved. That was the defining thought. After the breakthrough, I immediately started exercising that evening. Twenty-five years later, I'm still going strong.

People ask all the time why I still do it after all these years. I just stare at them wondering why they don't want to start.

That was the start of my fitness journey. Only now I'm not training for a race; I'm training for life. I'm training for those moments in life that you need to be strong to handle. You can't fake strength in those moments; life will call your bluff every time.

One crucial thing I have noticed in all those years of training is the most difficult part of this process is training your mind. That is why those rare, raw moments are so powerful. Once your mind is convinced of your renewed determination to overcome your fitness obstacle, your mind and body start working together in amazing ways to change no matter what life throws at you at any stage of your life.

Imagine coming home to see a letter and pictures of your adorable little girls on the table and the letter you are reading lets you know that your family will not tolerate years of my negativity and emotional abuse any longer. Sitting there alone in the house knowing they were ready to move on with their life without me was a wake-up call.

Those previous few months I was having a strong desire to question and wrestle the universal question of "is God real?" Having no faith in my life since childhood to my present moment of sitting in that house alone soon to be divorced, I was unaware that this would be the start of my faith journey.

Having so many questions about this so-called good and loving God and still not knowing the answers to what I needed to know to believe in him, I knew something life altering was about to happen. You know when you check the weather and you learn that a major storm is on the way. You notice that it's calm at the moment, but like it or not, it's coming directly at you. And if you're not prepared to take action, you will have to deal with the aftermath.

I knew I couldn't handle any more storms. I was done. I wanted freedom. I wanted to fully know this God that promises to love you despite all your messes and struggles, and not having it all together. I was tired, broken, exhausted and He was someone I was told who was trying to fiercely love me.

My family was begging for honor and strong leadership, the right kind of leadership. The type of leadership that once they see this strength and confidence they will gladly be a part of it, because they knew deep inside you have their best interest at heart. I started to put the pieces together. It was becoming clear once I knew what I was fighting for now.

Through tough conversation over the next few days, our family was now under the same roof again. Now with this renewed energy to strengthen our family, I embraced faith differently than before; I was more open-minded.

Our family life grew stronger as we went to church, and we started learning about how God is Love, and how we can learn through His teachings how to live an honorable life.

Now, as a doubter of faith most of my life and frustrated by the hypocrisy of the Bible and people in general, I wanted to be brutally honest with myself when I researched both sides of arguments for and against Him.

I'll discuss details in the next chapter, but there is an amazing quote by Maya Angelou that really sums up how it's possible to overcome doubt with faith if you choose to, not that this is a chapter to convert people; this is just my story and my experience.

This book is about finding this unknown strength that we have the potential of having, not a book solely on faith and finding it. If you believe faith is connected or needed to have this strength I'm referring too, that is up to you. But I promise you, my struggles with faith both past and present will be written about, and you will see for yourself if you relate or not to the struggles.

Continue being loving and be strong
Be fierce and be kind
and don't give in and don't give up.

Maya Angelou

Let me break down my thoughts when I started to apply what I thought she was meaning by those wise words. So first, what is love, and why should we continue to love?

Is it hard to continually love one another all the time? We all know the answer to that question. So is there really a way to love one another more than we think we could, or more importantly want to? We first need to know what love is right?

I read this beautiful description of love in this verse in First Corinthians 13:4-8. This description of love was told through divine intervention to a man named Paul.

"Love is patient, love is kind. It does not envy. It does not boast, it is not proud. It does not dishonor others, it is not self-seeking, it is not easily angered, it keeps no record of wrongs. Love does not delight in evil, but rejoices with the truth. It always protects, always trusts, always hopes, always perseveres. Love never fails."

What is so intriguing about this is he used to be a murderer of many people. He changed his life around instantly through divine intervention, and dedicated it to loving one another for the rest of his life, which he did.

Talk about a change of heart. It's interesting how someone once so evil could be responsible for sharing and preaching to everyone.

I know you can read that and think this world doesn't deserve that type of affection. Why should I care about a world so full of darkness that seems to seek and destroy people who care about others, and want to bring light to the darkness. The more painful thought is that every day we have the potential to share that level of love in one way or another to not only people we deal with every day, but also to the ones we care about the most.

An idea that really helps me try to honor my family is that this world definitely will not be a more beautiful place to live if we continue the same trend of treating people without respect and honor. We already complain enough about so much, either with other people's actions or the struggles that come our way.

We all crave the idea of our kids and loved ones being in a world that cares for one another, but we go on day after day just wasting a lot of potential away in one form or another. We need to show more action if we truly want to see this happen. Talking about it accomplishes little. Let me be clear, this isn't me being unrealistic or being soft.

I am a realist and logical person. I understand at some level the world will always have evil and hate in it. The only thing that has the potential to change it in any way moving forward is showing love and kindness to it, and yes there is a way to do this while being tough and strong.

If we want our kids and loved ones to experience any beauty in it, we need to start right now and live each day changing the world around us by our actions and creating this unknown and unseen butterfly effect.

This should be a very personal idea and high priority for you. People can easily be fake and fool the world, but you can't fool yourself. Once you have those brutally honest moments with yourself you actually want to be a man or woman of action. You want to live by your values and not worry about if the world is doing their part or contributing enough.

Perfection or obsessively trying to obtain all of these characteristics is unrealistic, especially all at once. Are there some ideas that may inspire us to be more aware of the world around us and show glimpses of love to others during our lifetime?

Every morning in this world, we can decide by our choices alone if we want to help change the world by aspiring to be the best you that you can and want to be. The other option is to stay status quo, and keep letting the same problems consume your thoughts over and over, and having the feeling of being trapped in your situation.

This was me, and once I reached a breaking point when I told myself I Want More, that was when my passion for change ignited inside. I wanted more out of life. Once I noticed that we are more connected together than we think, we all struggle and are looking to be noticed and be appreciated by others.

In this world we can all either do something or nothing. I had already done nothing; it doesn't take you anywhere in life. You stay status quo until death. I wanted to live a life whereas many days as possible I could say at the end of the day when my head hit the pillow "that was an incredible day." I know we all want that in our lives, and most people, including me, are unable to utter those words enough in our life.

Is it really that easy to literally just start being a better version of yourself right now even as you sit and read this? I couldn't be more serious when I say yes it is.

If you are truly frustrated, and you want to change and start living with a higher purpose and vision for yourself and loved ones, let's start right now.

Let's start showing those characteristics of love to everyone around us. Let's start living a life that you can look back on and be proud and smile that you lived honorably. And let's start living a life that shows strength and a life that people will remember you for exactly the way that you wanted to be remembered for.

I know you may be thinking that you are not in a good place to do that now. Start now anyway. I know you may feel that you don't have the resources or lifestyle to make a difference. Start now anyway. I know you will have this certain level of doubt, fear, anxiousness, and hopelessness that things will not change no matter what. Start now anyway, and don't look back.

When I started living and behaving toward my vision, I had a very vague plan. I thought to myself, "I'll just be as positive as possible all the time." Wow, how naive was that way of thinking?

Yes, we need to start on our vision right now, and not look back, but we definitely need to implement a short term and long term approach to pretty much all the choices that we make throughout the day.

Truth be told, this will be a humbling experience. At least it was for me. The problem was I was super motivated to start, but the next day something real hits you straight in the face—life. I thought with this new outlook on life, I would just pop out of bed ready to start the day, head to work, start being extra nice and making a difference with things there, and at home would just start aligning to my plan.

Yeah, that didn't work. I still woke up in the morning like a zombie. Being extra nice talking to everyone at work, I still had negativity still thrown back at me. The stress of paying the bills was still there. Errands still needed done running around town. Groceries, doctor visits, school events, etc., all stacked up. The to-do-list of life was still there despite your new awakening.

Do we just give up on our vision? Not a chance. In fact, those are the times we need to embrace it and become what the title of this chapter is: A new kind of strong.

If we just decided to live out our new visions, goals, and dreams, and then the next day use the same mindset to try to achieve it, life will retaliate against it. For some reason life likes to be difficult and set up roadblocks to stop you. That is the exact time you need to fight back the urge to give up. That is the exact time you need to say, "enough with that unproductive road". "I'm going off the road and off the beaten path to go around the roadblock."

It's time to be different, think different, act different. I'm hoping to help save you time, effort, and energy by exposing what did and didn't work for me.

First, to be different we need to address the normal stereotypes on certain topics so that we can learn how to move past them, and if you want, make efforts to possibly change the stereotypes by using your words and actions toward breaking the barriers.

I guess we will call it the "time to be different" breakdown. It was a wake- up call that I was so thankful to have. For the first time, I started to piece together all of the breakdowns I had over time. I saw a connection between all of them, and once I noticed this, I was able to put a plan together on how to fight life back. This type of new thinking was also the inspiration for writing my first book.

Since then, life has hit me even harder than I thought, forcing me to really dig deep after many private moments that included a range of emotions at different times from being super motivated all the way to being tired, broken and tears down the face. Those moments of vulnerability ironically helped show me how I now wanted to express strength and kindness to a world that consistently rejects it.

I knew what kind of man I wanted to be, and I was sick of the world how it was, and how I was allowing it to drain my energy and positivity sometimes to the point of borderline depression. I felt very conflicted on how I was living. It's when you live your life with an imposter syndrome, how you are perceived doesn't always mirror how you feel inside. You sometimes feel you have to take on the identity of what people perceive about you. On top of the world one day and then moping around the next. I would always be off track in some way either physically, mentally, or spiritually.

I noticed that two of the stereotypes that life camouflages the true meaning of, and the effect it had on the world was a huge factor on why I was failing at accomplishing some of my goals that I was struggling with.

Strength and Discipline were those two stereotypes. Once I embraced their true intentions, it ignited a new passion in me to first use them to change my way of thinking again, and this time change it for good. Once you have it in your life, you will never be the same.

The second was to write this book, and then show the world through my words and actions that it's a real change that you will be so grateful to have in your life. They go together to make this new strong be possible in your life. The world hates it because of its uniqueness, and it always inspires others in bold ways because it's so rare to see, and hard for the world to stop it because it defines stereotypes.

The first stereotype is Strength. I'm tackling this from three different viewpoints, but all three are extremely connected together, and come full circle in your life if you let it.

Physically you usually view strength as working out and getting those six packs and big biceps. The gyms are filled with mirrors, and people have no problem staring into it flexing and taking selfies to post on social media.

Hey, I was right along with them, and still catch myself from time to time. Now on the positive end of that, there is nothing wrong with flexing and looking to see your progress after putting in all that hard work. I've seen and have motivated myself also when someone has put in the work and they posted a picture with a positive message of staying strong and keep pushing those goals. It can give inspiration to many, and is a great way to keep in touch with others as you work on your fitness goals.

On the flip side of that, vanity is always ready to blind you to the true meaning of what is possible. Yes, you could post that gym pose of yours and caption it "Check out the guns." This is what hard work and dedication looks like." The other option is to post a picture of you helping someone out that physically didn't have your level of strength.

Maybe for example pushing someone in a wheelchair through a nature trail giving them a chance to be outside for once could be your goal. Giving them time out in nature and seeing Earth's beauty, whereas without your help they couldn't have experienced that. If people saw that post, maybe it would spark something inside of them to do the same, or maybe start working out so they could do the same type of community service that requires extra strength to be capable of helping out. It's all about taking your eyes off yourself and onto others.

The first idea of working out just to showcase your body is the stereotype we need to end. Flouting your body, and even worse, using your strength to bully others, is a problem that needs to end.

The new kind of strong I'm talking about here is using your strength, and instead of bullying, use it to stop it. Instead of flexing in the mirror all the time, maybe it's time to go out into the community and see if that strength can serve a bigger purpose.

That brings me to the spiritually part of strength. There are two characteristics that are at the core of how I want to be remembered for at the end of my life. I pray daily that I embrace both qualities together, and at the same time. Strength and Kindness. I know if you decide to use these two traits together, it will make huge positive changes in all areas of your life.

Just like above the idea of using your strength to help assist others that need it to take them through nature trails, do you see the beauty in choosing to inspire good in the world with your strength?

We all say we want to see kindness in the world. That's not going to be easy if we can't change how some strong people act in society. One of the ways to help change is to inspire others to try new ideas.

That means start working out and start involving fitness into your life so this renewed energy and mindset that you get from your new strength and new body can be used to show kindness to others and be different from society's usual stereotype of it.

A physically intimidating strong person helping others instead of bullying others gets people's attention fast, because people crave to be inspired. That is so rare. To see someone care for others so passionately but at the same time could take you down with one punch is fascinating to me, and very inspiring to me.

Mentally the only way to achieve this type of strength is to put in the hard work, which helps build a strong character. And people with strong character have the power to take on this darkened world. We must use discipline and strength the way it was meant to be used for. Many people aren't willing to change. They believe their life is just the way it has to be.

You must embrace every characteristic that most people view negatively, and instead view them as needed traits to become the new you.

As we move on to the other chapters, I feel I need to close this one with an urgent tone to it. Let me start by sharing this important quote that has shown me that it requires tough decisions and actions by yourself in order to make changes to you, and the changes you would like to see happen in the world.

"If you don't make time to work on creating the life you want, you're eventually going to be forced to spend a lot of time dealing with a life you don't want." ~Kevin Ngo

There is such a predictable pattern I have noticed when I talk to people who seem to complain, argue, blame, hate, bully, and degrade almost every person and/or detail of their life. Everyone and everything else is the problem.

The other predictable pattern I have noticed when talking to people who have a positive outlook is they accept the reality that life is not always fair, and sometimes it just plain sucks.

They also have seen love, beauty, strength, and kindness in the world. They realize that they are responsible for their actions and behavior. Then and only then will the changes you want to see happen.

We need to question ourselves more with our decisions, and see if our response to it will spark a change in us. Everything we struggle with can be taken with a more positive, more disciplined, and more strong approach. I know you will agree with me that we all want to see this world be the best it can be. We want to see love, beauty, grace, compassion, strength, and kindness revealed in everyone's heart.

Yes, I know it will never be 100% of the population, and others will tell you the same thing if you try to be a better person. It doesn't need to be 100% to make a difference though. Any action step toward positivity is a step forward in making this world and you thrive. Don't listen to others, though, if they are not ever trying to better themselves. They will never truly understand what you are thinking anyway. Just remember, you can only control your thinking and actions. Trying to control others' thoughts and actions is a lesson in futility.

We need to tackle every decision, every struggle we have about questioning ourselves. Are we taking the necessary steps and actions to push ourselves out of our comfort zone and trying different ideas until one of them sticks and changes are made? This will be consistently tough on a daily basis, boring at times, and usually goes against what society thinks is the way to respond.

Well, as a great wizard once said "We all must face a choice on what is easy and what is right." -Dumbledore (Harry Potter books/movies)

Get comfortable with being uncomfortable. Remember all of these traits mentioned above that seemed uncomfortable to embrace. They are now your best friend. They will always have the best interest at stake for you. They will never let you down. They will never disappoint you if you put forth the effort. It's blood, sweat, and tears time. Let's be a new kind of strong.

CHAPTER TWO

DESIGNED TO MAKE A DIFFERENCE

Ever heard the quote "Nothing changes if nothing changes?" Simple words, but the truth. Have you ever been in a relationship? It could be all your friendships with others, your spouse, your kids, co-workers, even yourself. That last one probably stood out, right? It always comes down to choices.

Once the other person(s) decides that they are not willing to dedicate their energy, passion, honor and integrity into the relationship, it starts to be impacted negatively and immediately. There is always this assumption that if they are in a close relationship with someone that they will always rise to the occasion, that they will never let you down. Well, we all have enough life experience to know that it is unfortunately unrealistic to believe that they will never let you down at some point.

Is it possible that we are in a relationship with a higher power who fiercely loves us but we are shutting it out or rejecting it? If that is true, you and the world are missing out on the greatest love story ever told.

A verse from John 4:13-14 explains "Everyone who drinks this water will never be thirsty again, but whoever drinks the water I give them will never thirst again. Indeed, the water I give them will become in them a spring of water welling up to eternal life".

Once you get a taste of what this higher power is talking about, you will want to change yourself and the world around you more and more. If you reject this relationship, all that could be will never be known to the world

We are only human, and humanity has emotions to deal with. Some are positive and some are negative. As a famous Harry Potter character once said: "We all have both light and dark in us. What matters is the part we choose to act on. That's who we really are."

I still want to be as transparent as I can when digging into this topic. This conversation needs to be honest with yourself, because as I have found out, it's extremely tough to move forward and make certain changes in your life until you find peace and transparency with this idea.

I needed to find some sort of answers to these questions:

1.Is humanity here on Earth without meaning or purpose? Are we just a freak accident? Are there no coincidences in life?

2. Was humanity designed to make a difference in this world? Are we connected to one another from something or someone we can't fully understand?

3.(Me being transparent and real) Throughout my life, even during times when writing this book. I have had random dark moments thinking of my pains and struggles, it seems maybe life is a mixture of both scenarios.

For instance, I deal with a lot of different types of people with my job. I can't tell you how many stories I hear of divorces, deaths, affairs, sickness, abuse from people sharing their stories that don't seem like they are part of some plan for good.

At the same time though, when I coached at Five Star Life and saw both coaches and students who are dealing with those same issues, but are coming together to share and help change their world together. I saw people making differences out of those random setbacks.

Society, either consciously or unconsciously, has been for years dividing people based on their beliefs and values. It's hard to find peace, clarity, love, compassion and grace when life and people around you are causing chaos around you everyday.

I was fortunate to realize in my early twenties that maybe life could be different than it looks in the day to day world.

This conversation is a must to have if we are to move forward with finding peace, and having a clear vision for how and what we will stand for. I know it's uncomfortable to talk about, but this book is about taking on the uncomfortable struggles in life and understanding that at the end of the tough choices we make after having all the options on the table we could find new direction with our life, we could find happiness by making the right choices for you.

I know that the two questions above spark many disagreements, and cause many to start debating many common topics that usually divide people into groups. Let me start by saying that I have always struggled with this topic. I feel for both sides of the arguments, not saying that to be politically correct and smooth tensions here. I already know I will not have 100% agreement on talking about faith or no faith.

If you really want to have a civil conversation about faith, or any other subject for that matter, you need to understand that your opinion, or your viewpoints, don't necessarily have to match the person you are having the discussion with. You could try to convince the other person until your face turns red with frustration that your viewpoint is the only correct one, but the bottom line is your opinion is your opinion. It doesn't necessarily mean you are right and the other person is wrong. It's just different. As long as the two of you can come to that agreement, it's possible to have a civil conversation.

When I was growing up, I did not go to church except for a few times when my aunt and uncle purposely exposed us to their church. I did like going there. Everyone was kind, and I was curious when I was there about this God they talked about. I never took it further than that level of curiosity as I continued to grow up, though.

The only "God" moment I had, and to this day was the strongest feeling and evidence to me about a higher power was during my field trip at school. I always noticed that I seemed to be at some sort of extra spirituality even without knowing God during the fall time. It is my favorite season by far, and even without faith in my life I sensed this connection I couldn't explain. During the field trip on a beautiful fall day in a moment of solitude around the barn of the pumpkin farm, I felt a brief wind blow around leaves creating this perfect autumn scenery. I felt for about a thirty-second trance this feeling I had never felt before.

It was this overwhelming feeling of love, gratefulness, and understanding that this beautiful fall scene I was in was a glimpse of a world that was fully complete. This world could be an amazing place if people chose love over hate. I felt I was in those 30 seconds living in a world full of love for the first time ever.

I did not want to lose that feeling, but it disappeared and has never returned to that level of serenity. Years later, when I decided I needed to finally figure out if I believed in God or not, I returned to that specific spot.

I needed answers to prove He was real, and since that was my big moment with Him, I thought He would reveal himself to me somehow. I felt nothing during that visit. I sat there thinking I must have just had some random feel- good moment back then. Scientifically, the brain is firing so many thoughts in your head 24/7 I didn't think God was responsible for that moment; it was just my feel good chemical reactions happening randomly.

The reason I tell you that story is because I do believe that was a God moment now. This is not to prove anything; it's just I know that we must look back on our lives, and then look in this very present moment and start making some decisions. The faith question must be challenged. Every human being needs to make a decision to either embrace it fully, reject it fully, or be open-minded until you are able to make a personal choice on how you will view life. Until that happens, you will have to follow your own path of faith and to allow God to be there as you traverse your own path through life.

You may decide to avoid the curiosity of faith, or just decide to not believe it. I was there in that mindset for many years. I lived day to day with this unexplained anger in me because I saw evil in this world—a lot of it. I didn't see things getting better, despite all these

Christians around preaching about solving world problems. I already had my explanations on how life was created, and how the universe was created, and how humans came from apes.

It all made sense to me then, too. I saw this evil happen in the world despite a God who says he loves people. I read a very confusing Bible that tried to explain life, and how we should live, but I saw people living and behaving in very animalistic ways just like our ancestors did.

I did try to be open minded about remembering moments in my life that did point to a higher power, despite what I saw in my day-to-day life. The first and most powerful moment was the field trip moment for me. I also had positive influences from my aunts' and uncles' attempts to expose me to their church in my early years.

In high school I was invited to a spiritual event, and for the first time I saw my close friends show me that there was a God directing them. I saw a friend's father lead a prayer as we all held hands in a circle around them. I felt surprisingly at peace with the idea of God even standing there, not knowing what to believe.

I watched a friend give up listening to certain movies and music immediately and started listening to worship songs instead. I was asked that day if I believe in God, and I said "I don't know." I was prayed for immediately, and I have to admit I felt this calmness as I left their house that day. It was a feeling of maybe there was something about this God.

After high school, one weekend I was visiting a friend in college, and we ended up drinking. We were walking the campus just messing around, and we walked up to a place that was known for people to pray. Even feeling tipsy from the drinks, I felt vulnerable and kneeled down to pray there.

In recent days I had been feeling extra frustrated and had this anger built up inside of all of my problems and struggle to find purpose in this world. I didn't know who I was praying to, but I just let it out that I wanted to find love, not only in life but find someone who I could love and would also love me back. Looking back on that moment, that time frame was when the questions and the need to dig into it was intensifying. What I didn't know was my prayers were answered but they were answered in a way that I didn't see at the time.

I would have never imagined roughly a year later living in my first apartment with my now wife getting ready to have our first child together. I asked for the opportunity for love which I was grateful to have in front of me. The bible says that love is patient, I'm grateful for that too because my newly formed family was patiently waiting for me to grow up and start being a man of honor and not a kid trying to get by life using his old lazy ways. Back to the point at the beginning of the chapter. If you are in a relationship with someone, and they are showing love, and you are not committed to them or have the same feelings toward them, you usually don't fully get it how much love is being shown to you. That was my relationship with God at the time.

What I also didn't know was that that relationship with Him is also connected to your relationship with your wife and kids. Which brings up to the moment from the first chapter where I was at a crossroads on how I was going to continue to live my life moving forward. This time I knew it was time to be serious about finding out what I was looking for in life. I acted swiftly about it like my life depended on it, because it did. In my mind I was going to start loving life or dive off the deep end.

This crossroad I was at was crucial to have in my life, because it woke me up. This awakening showed me not only the peace I was looking for, but it clarified the main struggles everyone has at some point in their life.

I knew my game plan on how I wanted to tackle this. I knew it would get personal, but I was ready to do this. Before I start this part, I want you to understand that my process of this game plan might be crucial for you to do in your own life.

My point in this chapter was to expose the complexity that society has done to faith. I wanted to simplify it. I researched this on my own. I wanted to know at the end of what I decided to believe that I could be at peace with it. I gathered all information on the support for God and also all the information against God. Through that process and piecing together my life's more spiritual moments and moments of darkness and pain, I found my peace.

Why this was important to me was once this process was done, I was able to understand the direction I wanted to go for myself, my family and loved ones, and how the world will be affected by it one way or the other. Whatever the outcome of your digging deep into it, your mindset toward life and with these questions probable will be tested in some way. These questions are a good place to start digging if you need a starting point.

Who am I?
What do I believe in?
What do I stand for?
Why am I doing this?
Who am I doing this for?
How will others be influenced by me?
What do I want to be remembered for?

Faith is such a unique thing. It causes wars and evil acts in the world to happen. At the same time, it solves world problems, and is responsible for many kind acts around the world.

For some, it is the problem in the world and people degrading it and rejecting it. For others, it is the source of all that is good in the world, and consumes their way of life to serve and love others

For me, besides a few unique moments in my life, that made me unusually curious. I pretty much rejected it. It took for me to be at an all time low emotionally and spiritually to decide which side of faith I was going to be on, and how that would move me forward. What I did know was that the path that I was on was staying destructive and consuming my emotions in a negative way on a daily basis, the cycle seemed endless.

Looking back now, I know this is something all people must find peace with, because it will start to consume your world sooner or later, especially when dark times arrive in your life, and I think we all know by now that darkness will happen to us whether we want it to or not.

I first looked back to see if I could find patterns of all the negative characteristics in my life, and then see if lack of faith was part of the problem, or if faith would be the solution. I grew up going to church a handful of times. My brother and I had biblical names but we hardly opened bibles growing up. Both sides of my family have an uncommon trait that everyone has been divorced or remarried. I mean everyone. So we both had preconceived ideas about marriage.

Two things I learned from that is not to take sides, and to hear both sides' point of view. That one would serve me well in life. I take that approach with many things in life, and it allows me to get clearer and trusting answers I needed to find out.

Unfortunately, I learned to be withdrawn more because I knew if I was vulnerable, and I showed my love to someone in a relationship that eventually they would get angry, and I would be hurt from the retaliation. Consequently, I would be scared emotionally. I definitely had trust issues.

Growing up, I spent a huge amount of my time sleeping in, playing video games, and watching a ton of TV and movies. I didn't have many restrictions on what I could watch, so you could imagine what teenage boys would watch and look at. Many things I watched usually had strong language, violence, action and nudity. There was easy access to Playboy magazines and even porn. I was just learning from my environment around me, and from family and friends what was normal to do.

In school, I learned all about how the universe was created, and how humans were created. We were just a freak DNA mutation from apes. Science books had all the answers. We didn't have cable then, and I liked to learn about nature and the wild, so any programs and documentaries that were on easily showed how nature was a brutal place, a fight for survival kind of place.

News channels consistently showed violent acts around the world and people committing crimes to one another. I couldn't help but see an eerie comparison between how the apes acted on the nature shows I watched and how people were behaving against one another, and the self preservation mode people were in. I thought to myself that we must be animals, because the evidence of the same traits we shared was undeniable.

It was a survival-of-the-fittest world out there just like in nature. Everyone seemed to be looking out for themselves. All of this media I was watching was before the internet and smartphones, so the choice for media outlets was limited to getting information.

On top of all the negativity that I did see going on, it seemed all the spiritual and church-going people were eventually shown in the spotlight on the national news as frauds. Committing crimes like child abuse, rape, lying, scheming and deception were always popping up in the news feeds.

It just solidified my belief that faith was nothing more than some fake way of making people believe in being something more. If it were true, and people really did make life changing commitments to this God called Jesus, then why did everyone who believed in him act the same as everyone else?

I thought He was supposed to be this life changing experience? I saw nothing but hypocrisy, and I knew that they knew deep down it was all nothing.

So this was my mindset for years, that all people truly knew there was nothing out in the world, no God. It didn't matter how spiritual they were, they knew deep inside the truth.

That was what I kept telling myself, when in fact I was struggling inside for years on what was the truth. I had some unexplainable moments in my life, but at the same time I felt comfortable with the idea there couldn't be a God.

So when I looked back at my life, some intense raw thoughts came into my head. I knew I needed the truth no matter how cruel it was to think of it that way, or that I had been deceived by society's influence all these years. The raw thoughts were these in my mind:

* We were all just a freak random accident in space, and just DNA mutations from animals on Earth. Our wants and needs as humans were similar to that of pure animal instincts, especially the apes. There is no God or anything else out there guiding us. There is no right or wrong. Like in the animal kingdom, this is a brutal place with random events happening.

*There still seem to be so many connections in nature that seem to be working together to form ecosystems and consistently changing life cycles that are working very well to make this planet create beautiful life. It has too many things working together in a world that is supposed to be a random chance of being here and life just accidentally being created here.

*Murder, rape, unexpected deaths, horrible deadly car accidents, random sex, lying, stealing; there were no acts of evil in this world, because evil doesn't exist. Evil is only talked about in spiritual books, and since those are fake, all of those things are just happening with no rhyme or reason, right?

*Even thinking those thoughts above, something deep within myself truly didn't believe that it could be true. That would mean no coincidences have ever happened. Every single thing is just by chance. I see too many coincidences in my life and in others to believe that it is all by chance.

*If there is no evil, then there is no spiritual battle going on in this world like the Bible talked about. I still see people fighting to change this world despite its bleak future and trying to change it. They are trying to change it through the teachings of a man named Jesus who lived thousands of years ago who many claim their life changing behavior is because of Him. These people are either literally crazy in the head, or they see something I do not. Either this Jesus is the biggest con artist of all time, or the greatest teacher to the world that it has ever seen.

*I could slightly relate that this loving God was not responsible for hate in this world. He was the God of love, right? If this darkness or Satan was scheming all this pain and hate in the world, why is he allowing such acts to happen? Even if these evil acts were not caused by darkness, and they were just random acts happening, God not stopping it was the same as you knowing someone was abusing your kid or loved one, and you had the ability to stop it, but just let it continue. Why doesn't God stop evil from happening when he has the power to do so is one of the most questions I see asked by people, including myself.

*While there always will be Christian hypocrisy around, the media always seem to be willing to expose the worst cases to families at home watching the news. Why are they always concerned with Christians more than any other groups about exposing them? If there is no God, and that is all a joke, why take so much time and effort to expose someone who is not real? I always wondered why do they consistently try to downplay His existence and power, so much time and energy and resources spent all to tell people not to believe in this man who lived thousands of years ago, and was supposed to be crazy, and just a normal man with no special powers. I also thought that if the Bible was right, and there was a spiritual battle going on, and one side was trying to stop the other, that these methods that society had in place to weaken one side's agenda were very effective. That also meant, though, there was an actual spiritual tug of war thing going on, which meant that something big was going on behind the scenes of the human race. The fight for creating people to strive to make a difference in the world, or setting up plans for total destruction was being created by an evil force.

So I know expressing my thoughts above are definitely debatable arguments. I know that many reading this may question my loyalty to my faith. I also know that more people have more detailed questions, and maybe have answers to some of those thoughts. I also know that every person on Earth has an opinion. I know mine are just as equally valuable others can relate to. My take on things, and then hearing my story, and then researching their own insight will open new doors on the direction they want to take their life.

So here is how I found my answers by researching those thoughts to figure out this whole "Is God real or not?" question.

*The vastness of the universe is so complex that it will remain largely unexplained exactly how or why it is doing what it is doing, and how long it has been growing, whatever it is growing in too. Much of space seems to just be randomly happening while other events such as the existence of Earth seems to have a plan in place and reason for existing.

A beautiful and unique planet like Earth I believe is accepted as a miracle for being in space surrounded by planets with deadly living conditions. While there can easily be other life forms in space, other life in space doesn't discredit that a creator had a role in our existence.

*I believe we are more than a random DNA mutation from primates. We do have very similar connections and similarities. The connections are so many that I find it hard to believe that people can flat out call science and the observation of evolution crazy ideas. I just don't believe the evidence is so one-sided that it is easy to figure out life's origins. I believe that

God created us, but the Bible is unfortunately confusing in my eyes about it. I'm sure that is for a reason beyond my demand for clear answers. The absolute is that God created us. The definition of evolution is change. Anyone can look around the world and see that nature and animals change to adjustments in their environment. It's happening all the time in front of our eyes. How is that evidence, though, of disproving the existence of God. God creating people and animals and ecosystems that are capable of making necessary changes to survive and make a better way of life is a vital God-given ability, and amazing characteristic traits to have. Did we come from primates? I personally don't think so, but similarities are there. I have come to peace that I will not have concrete answers on the beginnings of the human race, however it happened.

*My biggest issue with faith all these years is I know it's one of the most popular questions thrown in the face of Christians and people debating the existence of God. Why is there evil in a world created by a God of love? My question was lesser then that one, because God or not, evil exists. I always thought it was interesting that people debating God would bring up evil? The explanation of the existence of evil is found in the Bible in which they didn't believe in. My question was not so much as the evil part, because I truly didn't believe God causes evil to happen to people so he can prove how glorious he is in some agenda he has going.

For example, I don't believe He gives people cancer, or makes someone get in a deadly car accident, or have babies get some awful disease at birth to prove some point. My question was if He is in control of all things, including his opposite Satan, or as I call it, darkness, then why is He allowing power to him to create whatever scheme and evil acts which he is a part of every single time? He is given some type of control of this world, but no matter at what level I just don't understand. I know I'm not alone in this frustration. Even as my faith and relationship continue to grow with Him, it will always be my main frustration, and but no matter if He chooses to answer it one day or not, I will keep moving forward to help make this world better even as those evil acts happen.

*It was easy to believe that we came from primates when I have seen physical similarities that over time could become what we are today. I have seen people be just a savage as you see in a family of primates known in the present. I have seen anger and deceitfulness. I have seen people act just as a primate would with a toy or with food, full of a certain self-preservation mode of this is mine, and I will take and harm whoever tries to take from me. I have seen similar human approaches on their way of taking care of their needs as far as what seems to be the basics of survival--food, water, shelter, reproduction, offspring. I was also so blind-sided to observing one version of how people were acting in the world. Once I became curious, if people could be different from acting this way, it really started to open my eyes. Instead of thinking how much we are alike, I wanted to see the difference people were from them. I saw a connection to nature with people. Was there a connection to a higher power, which may or may not be related to nature?

I know the last few pages seemed like a venting overload of all the hatred and anger I had with faith. Please understand I just want to be honest with my thoughts. After years of digging into my faith journey, I started to realize that just because there were some connections and maybe some truth to the above statements about the problems with faith doesn't discredit it from existing.

I started a different mindset of thinking because I was tired of living with hatred and anger all the time. I wanted to find peace and wanted love and strength and kindness to be in my life.

I read a powerful quote by Nelson Mandela one day that read, "If we can learn to hate, we can be taught to love." I thought all these years of society designing life and our daily routines, maybe there was a different path to travel on. I wanted to start living a different way. I wanted to use whatever gifts and talents I had, and start helping the world out with them.

I became aware of all of these people who told me that you can't pursue those ideas, because there was no time for that stuff after working all day and trying to make a living and raising families. I felt like their minds were limited in their thinking about and what they could become. I wasn't about to let their limits be pushed into making me have them. I was in uncharted territory. I felt I was now growing and pushing the limits on what I was capable of taking on and learning about, the only way to find out how far this path was going to take me was to keep pushing my limits.

Someone told me that Jesus' purpose for us was to expand on what we already know and are good at, but to do something that you would have never imagined. I started making a game plan to change how I lived. I was going to start doing what I had to do, so I could do what I wanted to do.

The reason why most of these problems exist in this world that I was complaining about seeing was that while men were busy being evil in this world, the good men were doing nothing to stop them. We are too busy watching TV and playing video games. We are too busy working jobs we hate to make money to buy houses and cars that we can barely afford, and don't spend much time in because of all the work. We need to wake up from this nightmare and realize that we need to be who we really are in this world, no matter what this society says is possible and not possible. Don't settle just to make a living; start making a difference.

The chances that you take, the people you meet, the people that you love, the faith you have, that is what's going to define you. I had to dig deep to figure out this faith thing. It was like cancer. You can't just wish it away and just sweep it under the rug because it just lingers and stays there. You must deal with the cancer and figure out what is going on and take action. A higher power designed you to seek the truth throughout your life. The more we fight it, the more it just festers.

So, yes even still to this day I have many frustrating questions about faith and this world, but I have learned more and more each day that I need God in my life. Every single time I try to do life on my own, I end up needing Him to bail me out, teach me to be more humble, kind and show love in a way that I can never figure out on my own.

So again, strength is not optional. We need a certain strength that comes from our faith in our life if we are going to make a difference in this world. Sure, we can do some good deeds here and there and not believe in God. I endorsed those thoughts, and they felt good to do. I can tell you it is a night and day experience to make a difference in this world with God as your inspiration. The ripple effects of those experiences is something I hope I get to see in the full circle moment one day.

Is this my plea for you to become spiritual? I know better than most that everyone is on their own path. Faith is something that is prevalent in my life, because the starting point is where I changed paths. I wanted to stop evil that was causing weakness to this world, and in my own way start creating strength for this world, and to do that I would need a game plan, a design. So yes, I now believe we are designed to make a difference.

CHAPTER THREE

THE SOUND OF SILENCE

If I were to ask you what you are afraid of, what would you say? I looked up various websites and put together a top five for us to look at:

1. Public Speaking
2. Death
3. Heights
4. Scary animals, insects
5. Confined spaces

Now there are definitely some things on that list that make me nervous. Up until about two years ago, I would have agreed on that list. Now I believe there is a new number one on the list. Not giving it the respect that it deserves has cost my life so many missed opportunities. In fact, I believe if you do get time to enjoy this every day, it will change your life and create a mindset, so you could conquer most of those on that list above.

Silence. I believe this is the most feared thing in people's lives.

In defense of today's way of living, it would be hard to have silence in one's life. We have 24/7 technology news feeds of social media, news, entertainment, and screens in every direction to keep our eyes and minds so busy that our mind is in overload with all this information.

While all of this is hovering over us, as I said before, we are busy waking up to go to jobs we don't like, so we can buy houses, cars, and luxuries that we truly can't afford. We start the cycle over each morning, and meanwhile we daydream wondering when our big break will happen or when things will start to go in our favor.

Now, you would think that since everyone is so upset with their daily routine that they would come home extra motivated to pursue their passions and use their gifts and talents to help themselves, their families, and their community. On the contrary, it is quite the opposite. Society is also getting increasingly obese and addicted to more sugar, carbs, and stimulants in drinks more than ever. The food they eat is not providing the right energy, and they are coming home more tired since their sugar and caffeine high isn't lasting.

When the majority of people come home from all the chaos of their work and all that involves that, they also just don't have the energy to deal with much more, let alone take the extra time and energy to pursue their passions.

Now, don't get me wrong. I understand and have been guilty of doing all the above as well. I have a physically demanding job, and a high metabolism, and was still in good shape, but I was definitely off balance in the foods I ate. I would come home starving all the time, and checking my phone often also. I tended to put things off until the next day so I could have more free time to do what I wanted.

I hardly wrote things down on paper, so ideas and the fix-it list for the house would come and go in my head. I never prioritized much, so I was off balance on how much time to spend with the family, time to fix the house and car repairs, yard work, and errands around town.

Unfortunately, I know many people who live this way, and while their mind is wandering all over the place, they are wondering why it seems like there is always a to-do list to accomplish. They are also asking themselves when they will get more free time, but at the same time, while they are pushing off the to-do list, they are on their phones or flipping through cable TV. It doesn't take long for an hour to pass by...then two...then three. Stats also show that many people don't get the right amount of sleep (guilty here too).

So we push off all of the daily grind stuff, and we think we are getting the down time we deserve. In reality, however, we are adding to our list. We are not actually resting anyway, since our eyes are still glued to screens, and still lacking sleep time. That doesn't sound like the right game plan for life, does it?

Another eye opener for me is when (myself included) you ask someone what they did last night, and their response is "I was a little bored." Wow, that should be a huge wake up call. Let me be blunt, and take it from me who has said this before. If you are saying that in any part of your day, you need to reevaluate life ASAP. At the same time you are "bored," your relationships with your spouse, kids, friends, co-workers, even your pets are being deprived of your love. Instead of screen time or sitting around saying that, we should be taking that time being wasted and go make memories and experiences.

Go find your loved ones and spend time with them. It doesn't even have to be an all-day thing. Go to a movie, go get coffee and talk, take kids and the family dog to the park. Do something. Just use those hours and even extra minutes focused on how to make something happen out of that time being useful instead for life-wasting minutes that are disappearing forever.

Don't feel like too much time has already passed, or the damage is done already either. "The time is always right to do what is right," said Martin Luther King Jr. I read in many books that continuous improvement is always better than perfection. No, we can't change the past and fix mistakes, but we can start this very minute and decide to use our precious time for honorable memories.

We also can use some of that "bored" time to pursue passions or talents. Over time I have been slowly learning how much time, money, and energy is being wasted on things that should be considered low priority.

Even after I decided to never say I was bored again, I still had problems finding a balance. My work schedule was changing for the worst, and I was working more hours, and I still wanted to be able to get stuff accomplished at home. I started reading some books and magazines on how to be more productive. I thought I now had a game plan on how to change some things around, because like many out there I was ready for a change in my daily routine.

Now, I would come home and not waste time on screen time. I would take on a project that I thought needed done. I thought I was a good multitasker because I had stuff on my to-do list every day, and I was getting those things crossed off.

Looking back, I was looking at my life a little backwards. I remember a distinct conversation with my wife, Stephanie. She wanted us to have a little family time, because overtime at work had caused a great deal of stress. When you work what seems like 24/7, all the errands you need to do can't be done, because the stores close before you get off work. The house and yard work needed attention on those hours you are not working, right?

She asked me one day to spend the one day off I had with family and forget the to-do list. Unbelievably, that request was met with a tone deaf response. Those errands "needed" to be done on my only day off. We at the time had a wall picture quote that read "Live how you want to be remembered." She told me that the only thing my tombstone was going to say was "Here lies Jeremiah, he got sh#t done."

Wow, what a wake up call. That was like my head hitting a brick wall. This whole time I was thinking I was putting in the work hours to provide good paychecks and getting the to-do list done every day after work, thinking I was kicking butt as a family man. To my credit, both of those mentioned are a priority for taking care of a family, but if you put them at the top of your list, some prioritizing needs to be done differently ASAP.

I felt like such a failure, and it really opened my eyes. I wanted to be better. I had been feeling off balance, but I continued to do what I believed many people do every day. They put their work and to-do list too high in their lives. I know the logical people are thinking, "Now you can't live a life or afford it if you don't put in the time at work and daily schedule."

Yes, you need to put in the work, but if you give all your energy to a company, and put in little time for yourself and your family, you aren't really "living" anyway.

To give a unique perspective, Warren Buffet is a billionaire. While he has influence and power, his life will be remembered differently than let's say Mother Teresa. Her bank account was vastly different compared to Buffet's, but she is remembered for changing the world in drastic ways.

So what is the answer? How do you achieve that balance? Is there a way to find a purpose and a plan to change your life around forever?

I didn't want to be remembered for being too busy for my family, or someone who only cared about a to-do list. I want my legacy to be all of the inspiring characteristics. Loving, caring, honorable, fun to be around, humble, strong, kind, compassionate, patient, and forgiving. I started to think that those dreams and visions weren't going to be a reality in the future, and it made my stomach turn thinking that the opposite could happen.

How did my life get so chaotic and so distracted that I had no game plan on how to manage my life, and create this vision I had for my life? The simple answer was I needed to have silence in my life.

Addictions are at a record high. Prescription medicine is at an all-time high as well. Society is trying to run away from their problems by trying to find a quick fix. The common thread in this book if you have noticed by now is tackling the problems head on and turning your life around by confronting our struggles, not trying to bury them.

People are using medicine as a way out of their problems. The problem with that is that quick fix has consequences. Nobody is paying attention to the fine print on the back of the bottle that has a list of side effects that cause added stress and bigger problems that could last longer than the problems you already have. The quick fix is leading to bigger problems down the road, because we are failing to bring the problem to the light, and deal with it no matter how serious the problem.

In society we are free to choose our actions, but we are not free from the consequences of those actions. We need to start changing our actions so that every choice we make is going to take us in the direction we need to go in, because no matter what, those decisions are costly.

Making the right choices affect not only you, but your loved ones as well. Choices, like a ripple effect in water, spreads more into our future than we think.

A few years ago, I was watching a video and the rock band group Disturbed was about to perform a new song. It was a remake of a classic song the Sound of Silence made decades ago.

It caught my attention, because the band was dressed differently, and the music set and setting had a piano and violins and instruments not normal for their music. It has a serious, dark tone to it also, like he was going to sing it differently.

He started the song slowly, and just when I thought he was going to add his classic rocker voice to the mix, he started singing beautifully instead. I never knew he could sing like that. The song was a massive hit for them. The lyrics were the other important thing that stuck out to me. The song is about this person who in this vision was shown how people are just living life, and not living outside their comfort zone.

They have all these talents and ideas in their heads, and no one is really taking action. They are just living day after day keeping to themselves. They are staying silent. Another lyric says that "silence like a cancer grows."

Think about how powerful that phrase is.

People decide to keep to themselves, because it's just easier. You can avoid pain and disappointment from failure, and letting yourself and others down in the process.

The problem is even if you try to live life that way, just like cancer inside the body, it still is living inside whether you deal with it or not. It will continue to consume you until the point that you either have to take it on aggressively or decide to let it consume your body, and it takes control of your mind and spirit. If you tackle the cancer early on and not avoid it, you have a greater chance of living a healthy life. The more you wait and avoid the pain, you just set yourself up for more pain later on. You must face the truth. Now.

After watching videos and reading books on the topic, I finally took the step, and decided I would wake up earlier than normal for a week and just try the idea of being alone and in silence, and see what I think about and what ideas show up in that process.

I have to say I loved it. I felt so at peace and in control of my thoughts. I felt like I was really able to focus with my thoughts exactly what I wanted to work on myself. It was really all about me at that time. I knew I could set up a vision for myself and my family in a clear state of mind.

Most people think that silence is just this emptiness, a waste of time doing nothing. It couldn't be further from the truth. It is full of answers, and the way to find vision for your life. I started writing out all the areas of life I wanted to work on in my life.

Then, for each area I answered with a question. I wrote the why, what, when, how for every vision I had for my life. For example, when I decided to write my first book I wrote that down, and asked why do I want to do that? How will I start taking on the process of doing that? What is the purpose of writing it? What do I want to see happen with it? How would I feel if I accomplished it? What experiences do I want to have with it?

Answering questions for each of your visions you have written down is a crucial part, because the answers will be the motivation for how to keep pushing on meeting those goals when life throws curveballs at you, and sets up roadblocks that will try to interfere and potentially stop your new found excitement on trying to accomplish them.

When daily struggles and interruption of your schedule prevent you from taking action on your goals, remind yourself why, and what will happen if you discipline yourself just a little bit more than normal today, and work toward your goal and dream despite the obstacles of the day. Imagine yourself fulfilling your vision in your head and enjoying that feeling of accomplishment.

I also wrote down my emotions, and how I believe others think of me at this point in my life: as a man, a husband, a father, a friend, a co-worker, and as a human being to others. I wrote down all my positive traits, and how and why those were easier for me to be a part of my personality.

I also wrote all my negative characteristics, and asked why I struggled with them. Do I want to change them? How could I make changes to be a better man. What makes me have those traits, and what are the trigger reactions that make me respond that way?

Those types of questions force you to really think about who you really are at this point in your life, and more importantly, if and why do you want to change anything.

It is this type of introspection, this type of soul searching, that is difficult to process. Most people don't like to dig deep into their character for fear of what they will find about themselves. They don't want to admit they are fallible to themselves or to others.

I loved seeing everything on paper, seeing all my deepest thoughts on paper. I felt a sense of peace that I was finally going to make sincere changes, and had a way to move forward with everything written down.

I wanted to share a general idea of some of the actions I do in the morning, and some at night before bed. This has been crucial for me physically, mentally, and spiritually for me to have some form of control of my life. I wanted to wake up each morning and not focus on work, bills, and the daily super busy schedule.

I wanted to wake up and have some sort of routine that would eventually become my usual way of starting my day. Knowing that I took time to invest in myself each start of the day, I felt like the day never got the best of me. The busyness and expectations of each day wasn't able to stop me from these actions that I did at home in the morning before I even left the house.

A generalization of my morning is this now:

-Get up, bathroom, get dressed.
-Drink full glass of water (body needs it ASAP to start functioning right away).
-Stretch for two minutes.
-Breakfast-pack my lunch, drinks for the day.
-No news, social media, or anything negative to watch or read. Instead watch or read for five minutes something that only is inspiring or motivating or helps me learn about what I have been wanting to become moving forward as new me.
-I'm spiritual. I pray to God to lead me, so I can lead my family and use his strength as a model on how I want to live and help this world. I do this for a couple minutes.
-I meditate after praying for 30 seconds to one minute.
-I look at pictures on my phone that I saved to visualize my visions and dreams coming true. Examples: pictures of a certain house, cars, traveling, things to experience with family, role models, quotes, prayers, person who has accomplished the same goal you want to accomplish.
-I write down daily action plans for my day: what steps am I going to take to get closer to those pictures on my phone that I am visualizing, write out my schedule, errands, what are two most important goals I am trying to meet now. I make sure no matter what I work on, I don't want my day to slip away.

In the spirit of transparency, I noticed one thing that I was disappointed to not see change. I still had problems getting immediately out of bed. My mind did seem to want to focus on being more positive in the morning, but only after a couple minutes of dragging my feet to shut the alarm off.

I still woke up, and the first minute as you all know, I felt negative because I heard my alarm from across the room, and knew the only way to shut it off was to get out of my warm comfortable bed and shut it off, especially before it starts waking my family or pets up from the noise.

Waking up in the morning has been such a huge problem for me all my life, and I thought that after reading all these positive steps on how to conquer my morning it would get a lot easier.

Well, not the first five minutes for me, but I did start snapping out of it quicker, and that time difference totally changed the way I started my day. I now understand that I will usually have a difficult time waking up for the first couple minutes. My mind is desperately trying to tell me to just lay there and go back to bed, don't start the day. It would be so easy to just lay there and start worrying about all the problems you have and how busy the day is going to be.

I have noticed that if I just make that decision to just start moving and get that alarm shut off, that tired feeling and that voice that keeps saying "just a few more minutes of sleep" goes away much quicker. I don't know what it is about that feeling and how your mind just wants you to lay there, but it's a strong feeling for sure. I now consider that feeling a roadblock that is trying to stop me from pursuing my dreams.

I know every day it will suck to do, but I just need to get out of bed as quick as I can. I know now that the quicker I do this, the faster that terrible feeling goes away, and just like that I feel awake and have started my day up early. The hardest part of my day is over, once I dispense of the unwillingness to jump out of bed.

After all the books and videos I have watched of people who have achieved many of their goals and dreams in their life, they all have this in common. They all get up early, and they have a morning routine of things they do every day. Everything about their morning is purposely planned out to prepare them to be successful in their day as they get started with it.

I have learned so much from others on this routine of setting up ways to help them not only wake up earlier, but ways to start your day on your terms. In my opinion you must embrace some of these ideas at some level to start your day if you truly want to make changes in your life.

Remember, this book is about taking on life and dealing with what needs to be dealt with, no matter how uncomfortable it seems. Everything that you want to see happen in your life is on the other side of those uncomfortable feelings, and those action steps that seem so hard as we do them on a daily level.

Here are some of the ideas that I have seen and read about many people who have achieved their passion and goals. These are random ideas, so take what you think will work best for you, and start some trial. Eventually, you will come up with a routine that works best for you.

-Get five and a half to seven hours of sleep. They pray, stretch, and journal as a night routine to help calm down and relax a half hour before. No phones, tablets, computers in the bedroom. Their room is very dark and set up so they are comfortable sleeping during the night. They set two alarms to wake up. They have also set out either their work clothes out or their workout clothes out so they have everything they need to leave their bedroom quicker.

-Drink a full glass of water in morning, eat a healthy breakfast, get healthy lunch, drinks, snacks ready to go for the day.

-Pray
-Exercise or practice a sport
-Visualize and meditate
-Run, walk, some form of cardio
-Read positive books
-Stretch
-Journal or write an action plan out for day.
-Spend time with family

There was a period in my life when my work schedule was getting so demanding that it affected my life at home both with my family and with myself. Now I know that is a big warning sign that it's time for change. When you wake up already worrying about work and bills and the growing to do list, it's time to try something to fix it before it consumes your life.

Since I couldn't adjust any time once I left the house, I knew all my hours were going to be used up by work, errands or family stuff. I decided after reading a book about changing your morning routine, I discovered it was much easier to invest in yourself. Life wouldn't be able to fill up your hours, so you have no time for yourself. Get up earlier in the morning, and use those hours to hammer out all your ideas and goals and dreams.

This is a huge deal to do. Yes I said do. I now firmly believe that you must choose at least some of those ideas above to put into your morning hours. This is to help you in your life, not give you more things to do in the morning. Remember, discipline is your friend, not something that is trying to rob you of more sleep by waking up earlier.

I actually was thinking wrong about this in my early stages of trying these ideas out. I understood that it was going to help me succeed, but I still thought of it as extra work that was going to pay off at a later time.

Another big problem I had, though I was getting up earlier with no problem, was I never adjusted my night routine. I was staying up longer than I should have. In essence, I was actually getting a little less sleep. I did like trying out new ideas in the morning but I was so sleepy I couldn't fully enjoy it. I would get the routine done, and finish my work day, and by the time I came home I was ready for a power nap.

Most of the time it barely took the edge off, and it threw my night off. I talked to my family about it, and knew it was time to finally make a point to go to bed early and get 6-7 hours sleep.

I also noticed a huge change immediately. I felt more positive in the morning waking up. I was thinking more clearly. I was more productive from the start. I still came home tired, but I was able to bounce out of it, and get my second wind once I ate and regained energy.

Isn't it funny how we keep pushing off sleep till the last minute of the day. We feel that once we go to bed, the day is over, your free time is over and you have to wake up and go to most likely a job you are now very fond of.

We would much rather watch that extra Netflix show, or be on our phones for an extra hour than give in and use that hour for sleep. We push past our tiredness and continue to do what we think is showing life's boss, and saying that we are strong enough to give up the recommended amount of sleep so we can do the things we want to do instead. We are not going to let life pass us by sleeping. We think electronics and screens are the answer, so we stay up later and keep our eyes glued to them instead of shutting them off.

How many of you can relate? I used to get up at the very last minute and scramble to get ready for work. I probably had four or five hours of sleep the night before, because I thought I was making my day last longer by fighting off my tiredness and staying up close to midnight.

I thought I was letting life pass me by if I went to bed at an earlier hour, and not being able to do whatever I was doing at the time, which, by the way, was non-productive most of the time.

Now the question to ask is how many of us wake up in the morning completely exhausted, and we told ourselves every day that we would do anything to be able to go back to bed and sleep?

Isn't it funny that the night before sleep was the last thing on our mind. After being so sleep deprived, your mind shifts to laying your head back on the pillow and catching a few more Zzzz's. You're just fooling yourself. Why are we putting off what we all know we need to do which is go to bed to get at least six or eight hours of sleep?

We think we are getting more freedom by staying up longer, and doing our thing, but the reality is that we just obsess about sleep all day long. We drag ourselves around and make countless mistakes throughout the day because of our tiredness.

This is backwards thinking. I remember my wife telling me instead of me coming home and trying to take a power nap she said I should try to re-energize. Why not go to bed at a better time. She was tired (pun intended) of seeing me drag my feet home, and instead of seeing her, trying to lay down for a nap.

She asked me why I never went to bed at a good time, so when she saw me, I would be in a better mood and not be so tired all the time. She told me she would have much rather have seen me go to bed earlier and not spend as much time with her. It would have eliminated obsessing about sleeping all the time. I ended up most of the time regretting laying down, because I had a hard time waking up from them anyway. It was a never-ending cycle of futility.

This is another area in which discipline is needed to change our lives around and give us a better life. It's time to change our mindset on this idea of thinking you can cheat your sleep schedule and brush off sleep. We need to get the sleep we need and use our awake time as honorably as we can because we know how precious and limited the awake hours are.

I think it's time to really show the power of making silence a top priority in your life starting immediately, like the next morning after reading this book. I think it is important to note that silence is not the direct answer to taking steps in dealing with what needs to be dealt with in your life. It's the starting block, and from there it will spread like wildfire into other areas in your life.

The direct answer is you, and the choices you make in everything you do. You will have a hard time deciding what honorable choices to make, though, until you take quality time first thing in the morning in silence. In the silent time, you are able to dig deep and decide what are the priorities in life today? Am I going to get uncomfortable today and take on my struggles, and also use my strengths for bettering my life?

You see, in the silence comes the answers needed to start moving forward. Let's say, for example, that you are struggling with your health and fitness. You may say you are overweight. So, you take your first 15 minutes of the day and write down the steps you will take questioning why you are overweight. In that time, you find out the reasons and then write action steps (big steps or small steps). I know life tells you that your day-to-day life needs to be go...go..go. Imagine the calming feeling I had that you control life's speed more than you think.

Everyone's life speed is different. It doesn't matter if you are taking huge aggressive steps or just trying small steps every time. You are still moving forward, and that is what counts. So say you chose to take small steps toward your fitness goals everyday during your new morning routine. You decide to dedicate

30 minutes in the morning to fitness time. You spend 20 minutes working up a sweat, and then spend 10 minutes looking up new exercises to try, or you look up new meal/snack ideas to help with the nutrition part.

You notice new ambition to wake up to invest in yourself before work even begins. You start noticing changes in your body after being routine with the new workouts and food ideas. You leave the house in better spirits because the workouts are making your energy levels higher. You are being more productive at work, because exercise is a natural stress reliever. Since your productivity is up because of the energy level, you get a raise. The new confidence in the way you look and feel, plus the new income is making life at home better, and the family is taking notice. Everyone seems to unconsciously be hanging around each other in the home more, because the positive energy is inside the whole house.

It all started with this impactful decision to be silent. Now, for all the haters out there who say it sounds too good to be true, and not everything plays out that easy, you need to be thinking outside the normal mindset that society trains us to be like, but there are valid points that need to be mentioned, because this is a book about being real with yourself.

The first point that I will make is that this workout idea really does work, because I have tried it. I have seen so many additional benefits from the workouts, and how it overflowed into other areas in my life. If you have read my first book, "Faith Family Fitness," you will know how passionate I am about how fitness naturally flows into your life to give you more clarity and vision for your life.

The valid points are that anything worth pursuing in life requires uncomfortable moments and choices. It sucks that it works that way, but it is what it is. As hard as that is to accept, the sooner we accept it, the better and easier it is to move forward, and start working for what we want to get out of life.

So on that note, yes, making a choice to work out every morning, and to research nutrition, or any other morning routine idea that we talked about trying is not always fun to do super early in the morning. The days where you are extra sleepy or flat out don't feel good, but you push through anyway is tough to do physically and mentally. The reward for that type of mindset though is very rewarding. Look at how the example of pursuing fitness goals flowed into other areas of life naturally.

Remember, during the rough times in the morning investing in yourself, I didn't know that it would start affecting other areas like that. That is the part I would like you to remember though. It's the unknown. You can't see it right away, but the sooner you see the discipline pay off, the more you want to see more changes like that and are willing to put in the work.

The alternative to not putting in that type of work ethic and discipline is a lot easier and more comfortable to maintain, but not very inspiring or doesn't put passion in you to love life. Like me, most likely if you keep the same routine of not being in silence you won't be able to listen to your inner thoughts, and also influence from a higher power.

You just stay in the trapped feeling the routine of wasting life away just working, paying bills, and letting days pass you by.

Of course, that way is slightly easier in the morning of just waking up, grabbing junk food for breakfast and scrolling through social media. You then find yourself being disappointed afterwards like most people either upset from seeing others succeed, or upset because you debate social issues on your news feed, and you let the responses anger you. It's a maddening circle of frustration, because it sets the tone of the day as you leave your house.

People all over the world are constantly trying to find shortcuts to help them be more positive, more fit, or be more productive everyday. I was one of those people. There are no shortcuts in life. I can be transparent with you, and tell you that it sucks a little and wish it was easier, but life is designed that way, like it or not.

You want to hear something crazy, though? I don't want to go back to the old lazy days after getting a taste of what discipline has to offer. As tough as it is, it really is like your best friend. It's always reliable, and has your best interests at stake.

It tells you exactly what it takes to get what you want, and if you put the effort it will give you not only what you want, but change you from the inside out. As easy as it is to avoid it, I swear it gets easier as you accept the work needed for your goals, because it changes you when you accomplish things in your life that you didn't think were possible to achieve.

It doesn't sound so crazy to invest a small amount of time each day to find answers to your problems and struggles and goals. That small amount of time turns into creating opportunities and creating habits needed to get you to that man or woman you always dreamed of becoming. But sometimes we lack the courage to push ourselves through life's barriers that always showed up in our face.

To close on this chapter, just imagine the unknown possibilities from you becoming this amazing man or woman, finding your passion and strengths through your self reflection.

I mentioned the song, "The Sound of Silence" earlier in the chapter. How amazing would life be if you could break through that type of silence? When people decide not to share their gifts, the world suffers. How amazing would it be to be able to share to the world your gifts and talents? Could all this happen because you one day decided to drown out the noise of life and just be silent for a moment? I am in awe of how powerful such a simple idea can be. Let's help ourselves, our family, and the world by being silent.

CHAPTER FOUR

ONE THOUSAND CUTS

Over 1000 years ago, the Chinese had a very unique and brutal way to punish and torture people till their death. They called it "Lingchi" or "death by a thousand cuts."

They would use a knife and make very small incisions throughout the body, one cut at a time. It was a very slow and painful way to die. It was outlawed years later, but unfortunately random cases still appeared from time to time.

Now what does this description of a brutal way to die have to do with improving your life and being helpful in your present life? Well, nothing, but there is a metaphor I want to use with this. Bear with me. I believe this metaphor will be crucial to apply to your life, and hopefully will be a huge wake up call to make changes now rather than later.

This metaphor popped in my head while I was researching habits. What makes a habit? Why are habits hard to break once established? How did we get good habits and bad habits in our lives?

I remember reading that habits can slowly form without one really noticing they are forming. One day you start doing something, then the next day, and so on. Usually they ease their way into your life, and you usually don't even notice over time. Before you know it, even the bad habits, you are overweight, addicted to something, or in a bad place mentally that seems irreversible to correct.

It's frustrating how easy and clever habits slowly start from being a "no big deal" to "dead-end roadblocks" in most people's lives, including mine. I know myself, and others, have to own up to the idea that we just can't let the same old habits continue in our lives. It's equally frustrating how some people know about those bad habits, but just keep on doing the same thing, knowing one day it will catch up with them. What makes them so powerful? Are we willing to sacrifice our true potential for some meaningless behavior?

The one thousand cuts method suddenly seems to explain habits and the effects of them very well.

Let us use this metaphor to explain how powerful some of our habits are.Take a few minutes and be extremely honest with yourself. What are two habits that have control of you right now? Are you having some trouble thinking which one is worse than the other? Are you having trouble figuring out which one has more control? The one that really fights back in your head is the one you justify that is not really the problem, that it's no big deal. That is your big one.

So when you are going over the habits, it's the one that says, "Anyone but this one" or "Surely not this one, because I love it" or "Are you kidding me? There is no way I can quit that." The harder your mind tries to justify the habit, or says that it really won't make a difference if you quit or not, that is exactly the one that has control over you now.

Another honest conversation that needs to happen is what is the hidden motive of the habit that has control of you? For me, I took it very personal once I discovered that my habits would be formed both directly and indirectly from society.

After years of self doubt and figuring out what I believe, I made the decision that I was in the middle of some sort of war with myself.

Let me explain.

While researching my spiritual curiosity, I discovered two things I now believe in. One was no matter how confusing religion and God was, I couldn't brush off what I saw in this world, which was at some level a battle between good versus bad or light versus darkness. As crazy and as dark as this world can be, I have witnessed or have been a part of beautiful moments that proved to me that part of the human race, and part of the world are here to protect and honor this world.

Unfortunately, part of the human race and world are part of darkness and have no desire to change it for the better. My faith is in Jesus, who I believe stops weakness, and creates greatness in you.

I totally understand and really do respect people if they choose to believe in Him or not. After all the years of struggling with life and also seeing and knowing what I know about him through the world's eyes, I can see how people need to find their own answers about him.

I'm sorry to bring this deep conversion up again right before we discuss our habits. I bring it up, because once you figure out what habits need to be dealt with, it helps to know if they involve your spirituality.

So here is where we are. We have discovered what habits need to be dealt with in our life. We then figure out how impactful they are through spirituality. Are they impacting not only us but others and our future family members generations?

Remember, a lot of these bad habits will get passed down to our next family generations either through DNA genetics or through our children watching our actions, and habits and copying them either directly or indirectly when they start to live their lives. Sadly, these two powerful ways to pass things along continue to destroy a family's potential.

It's time to do something mentioned in the Bible. It's time to call you out of darkness and into God's wonderful light.

I brought up those two debatable issues of God and spiritual battles, because I believe these habits are crucial to bring out into our personal conversations we have with ourselves. They not only affect you, but your family and your potential to be a light in the world, if you believe in that or not.

Society has done a great job of hiding our dangerous behaviors. After all, look at social media. Scrolling down your newsfeed, no problems to see here. All is good, all is positive, and everyone seems to have fantastic relationships, and everyone seems to be on vacation.

The first part of this metaphor we need to do is acknowledge the process:

1. Admit you are being cut (have bad habits)
2. Stop the cuts (find solutions/take action to stop)
3. Prevent the cuts (preemptive steps to avoid re-cuts)

So if you have thought of some bad habits or "cuts," you already have mental toughness. Most people are just surviving on "auto-pilot" and let their mind take control of the majority of their thoughts. I don't blame them, because I am a victim of this too just like everyone else. It's something that we can never fully stop from happening, but we certainly can control more than we think.

You may also be thinking what thoughts are real and what thoughts are being auto-piloted. To be blunt, habits that make us feel insecure, unworthy, weak, fake, angry, frustrated, depressed are the ones that are our darkness. They disguise themselves as the answer to the problems of life. They make us feel comfortable when dealing with uncomfortable moments in life.

I know it's tough and humbling to admit that these habits are the "failures" of our lives, and the choices that keep us from going the direction we truly want to go in. It may seem like we have a choice to just stay the same, and tell everyone to mind their own business. This book is about bringing out the darkness. This is about understanding that know matter what you decide to do, one way is an easy way to live, and the other is harder, but will lead to a better life and a better you.

Either way, you are going to feel the consequences of your choices. As JK Rowling beautifully said: "Some failure in life is inevitable. It is impossible to live without failing at something, unless you live so cautiously that you might as well not have lived at all. In which case you fail by default."

Wow, let's start to stop pretending that these small "no big deal" cuts to ourselves are meaningless every time we choose our habit of destruction, or eventually the cuts will become our one thousandth cut, and the final cut is made.

Every cut is making an impact on us. It's time to stop the bleeding.

When I was ready to start making some changes in my life, I researched many websites and watched many YouTube videos on people who have made many drastic changes in their life. I took on the info I saw and heard and put together the top five most common and helpful ideas to help make choices that will help you in your life. Let us find out what we truly want.

1. Be You not Them – It's time to stop worrying what everyone is doing or saying on social media and in your daily environment. I don't care what people are posting on news feeds. Everyone has problems and struggles in some form or another. Some people just hide it better than others, but we are in the same boat, I promise you. You show the world by your actions (not your words) what you stand for. I believe deep down everyone is looking to be inspired by someone who is not fake, but is sincere, humble, strong, and kind to everyone. Someone who has honorable characteristics and makes you smile when they think of them..be that person.

2. Fight for what you want – You need to understand that in order to make these changes, you will encounter obstacles, roadblocks and be forced to make quick and uncomfortable decisions that could compromise your new habits you are trying to make a part of your new mindset.

When boxers train for a fight, they train daily very aggressively and have a clear objective with each workout they do. Every choice and movement is to train their body and mind to be disciplined enough to take the pain, and no matter how tough that current moment is, they prevail. Maybe they are having a tough day or an injury to deal with. They push through knowing that the pain will pass, and they have to push through the uncomfortable feeling in order to get to their goal.

That is how you need to approach your choices that seem to be so hard to keep years of bad habits from reappearing. These new habits and ideas will not stand a chance without your fight for them.

3. Know what you want and focus on it – The first two ideas make you first get real and raw with yourself about who you truly want to be, your belief system and your character. The other shows your determination, and how willing you are to change yourself. Now you need to get tunnel vision and keep focused on what is important to you on a daily basis.

Remember, every day life will throw curve balls at you to derail your new habits and beliefs. Let us remember that no matter what life throws at you, our attitude determines our direction. Don't focus on the moment, and let your first immediate emotion control or change your beliefs.

Pretend that you will have to play a video of your responses to your family later on. Will it still show your true and authentic self? Remember that everything good and bad passes quickly. Stay focused on the new you.

4. Always be prepared--One thing I noticed in my life is that no matter how strong my faith was, or even when I didn't believe in having faith, the darkness of this world is relentless.

I, nor the world, have many concrete answers about the power of it. It sucks, but this supernatural sort of force is strong, and believable in my opinion. I know you see it too at some level. That is why I agree with the others who we need to be prepared to defend our character, good habits, and everything we believe to be honorable in our life.

Every day society, people, and random events seem to work their influence on us. All the negative aspects of life rub off on us, and sneak negativity on to our mindset.

We must create a "shield" around us to block as much resistance as possible from the outside world, so our values and habits will continue to grow daily. Your thoughts, as powerful as they will become over time, will always be vulnerable at some level caused by some random unexpected moment or person.

Some of the ways to help cope with this is to do a few things. Start with your phone. We are all on it way more than we need to be. All of your social media connections should promote positivity. Anyone or any connection that promotes hatred, divide, violence, close-mindedness, should be dealt with by hiding, unfollowing, snoozing, deleting, or blocking.

It shouldn't matter if they are friends, co-workers, or family. You choose the best method to limit their impact on you, but this needs to be done. If you are having a hard time deciding which people to limit in your life because it looks like almost everyone is your friend,

read this quote. "Understand people by their actions, and you'll never be fooled by their words."

I have learned so much about people this way. It actually sucks to think about it, because I have been let down so much by many. Sometimes, though, the best way to deal with some people is not to deal with them at all. I know we all have those people in our lives now.

It sucks, but those people and personalities will always be around. Avoid them at all costs. I have also been surprised by others, though, and their commitment to me and my family. I know that will be a helpful tool to use to decide. Limitations also go for entertainment too. If you feel that these forms of entertainment are harmful for the success of you and your family, limit them immediately.

This may include certain types of movies, music, night clubs, sports bars, websites, dating, and screen time. Of course, I'm not promoting living a boring life or being a super serious person all of a sudden.

Use your fire-in-the-gut instinct and common sense to decide what should go and what is tolerable, and what can stay for now.

Remember not to be hard on yourself if you slip up or let emotions or people get the best of you sometimes. There is no perfection; life is life. Do your best and move on from it in the most honorable way you know at that moment.

5. Do things out of love—Now, that is a powerful statement. I truly believe that if we can put this into action in our lives, everything and everybody can live in such a beautiful world. All of your new mindset and habits and rituals should now be associated with love. I

know it is a tall order, and easier said than done in some circumstances in our lives. I know hate and darkness consistently trying to reverse the positivity we try to create for ourselves and the people we love.

I remember many times trying to be the bigger person, and trying to possess all those positive characteristics to everyone only to be screwed over by someone or something. I started to doubt that love could change things in this cruel world. I thought it was easier to be realistic and be in self survival mode all the time.

Do you know where that road leads? Nowhere. I remember many times coming to a "mental crossroad" and decided which course to take. I remember thinking my normal way of doing things always lead to the same results-- Hate, boredom, predictability, anger, rage, and more frustration. I think to myself now in those moments when making choices that I have already chosen that path before, and that path leads to nowhere and feels like death.

I try my hardest every day to do things out of love now. Do I fail to act out of love while living in this world? Absolutely. Life is tough, but you already know that. I do know that I haven't come this far in my life without embracing those ideas mentioned above.

Being me and not them. It's about me humbling myself, and realizing I don't have it all together, and that is OK. It's about me questioning myself and being raw and real about who I truly am, and what I want to show the world is who I am. To be in a fighter's mode about handling life and showing the world that no matter how tough it is, that I'm willing to fight for my beliefs, values, and what and who I love is what is most important.

It's about watching out for the resistance of this world, or the darkness. It's important to understand that no matter if we want to change ourselves or not for this world, this force is out there, and it is nothing but death and destruction. There is no love associated with it. If you feel any part of you or your life has this feeling of anger, hate, death, and destruction, it is time to fight back. That is exactly where you start making changes, no matter how uncomfortable and humbling it will be.

In fact, if it does feel like that, then get even more serious about those changes. Remember, anything done out of love will have resistance to it, like it or not.

I'll end this chapter by showing my general blueprint on how I try to live my life, even as I write this chapter. I concentrate on these two characteristics because I feel that if they are done correctly, they represent love. If you are feeling lost right now in life, and feel you don't know where to start making changes, maybe start with these two ideas. If you are familiar with my first book and social media, you know that I embrace those two traits in my life, and try to live by them.

Be Strong
Be Kind

Physically—Start or change your fitness perception to understand that you need to be in the best physical shape for your current moment you are in. Life is tough. I know what some of you may be thinking. "I'm not in your shoes." I don't know the handicaps and injuries and heritage and background. I don't know your daily time schedule. I know time is hard to come by, and there seems to be more important things to get done before worrying about being fit.

People can tell me all day long their excuses, but they don't convince me they are OK with not being fit. Everyone thinks about their body every day wishing for better results, but there are many excuses to pull out of their hat to use for the day (some may even be valid ones).

I don't need convincing. Fitness has changed my life forever. You need to sit down and figure out what needs to change now. You want new habits and ideas to live by. They will be extremely hard to keep in your life if fitness at some level is not involved.

Find a doctor for a check up, find a fitness mentor to see how to get started. Find a workout partner if you need social support, but you just need to start and get movement in your fitness life. I promise changes in all areas of your life will start to change.

For those of you who are already in shape and know how fitness has changed you forever, share those experiences and passion with others. Be uplifting and help others who are weak.

Show them kindness; show through your strength that power and strength can be used to make the world a beautiful place. Use your newfound strength for positivity around the world. Be humble.

There is a fine line between cocky and confident, though. Embrace your new body, and be proud of it, but always stay humble. If you look the part, you will not need to convince them. Your strength will attract and inspire others if done right.

Mentally—Being strong mental is attainable if you apply many of the ideas mentioned in this chapter. Once you start keeping fitness a high priority in your life, the benefits from the exercise are encouraging to say the least. Your mind will be fueled by all the nutritional items you are now consuming to maintain that new body of yours. You will have more clarity and focus when making decisions.

Keep your mind strong by keeping the body strong, and feeding your brain with the right fluids and nutrients needed to thrive and help you make better decisions. Read and journal more to keep your mind thinking and staying sharp.

Keep as much negativity away as possible, and don't cloud your mind with harmful words and thoughts that happened during your day. Make kindness a priority for one of the ways to help keep a strong mind.

In everything you do, train your mind to embrace kindness by having everyone and everything be as positive as possible. Stress will eat you alive if you let it. Negativity is in everyone's lives all the time, including me.

I'm not saying to pretend it doesn't exist and "just be positive." I understand the difficulty of what I just asked you to try to do.

It will never be 100% accomplished in one's life. That is one of the points, though. Since we know it will always be around, we need to be as strong physically and mentally as we can to stand a chance.

Speaking of standing a chance, if we are dealing with some sort of resistance or dark power or energy, we need guidance from a higher power or energy to also have a chance.

Spiritually—Every day, especially in the morning before I start my day, and set the tone for the day, I try to do at least one of these things: Pray, mediate or at least take a couple controlled deep breaths. Read, journal, jot down notes about your goals and dreams. It's important to put into existence the thoughts you want to achieve for you, your loved ones, and how you want the world to see you. Just thinking and asking for things, though, is not the right path for the answers you are looking for.

I pray knowing I am willing to put in the blood, sweat, tears needed to accomplish my goals, dreams, visions, and overcome all the obstacles that will be there to second guess my determination to get there.

Stay strong and show kindness spiritually by spending honorable time with your family and friends often. Stay strong and show kindness to the circle of people who you deal with in your daily world. Make time to be outside and enjoy and soak up the beauty of nature. I promise you being with people you care about, and also being outside in nature will bring clarity and refocus you every time. I promise you if you make a point to be in nature, and even better with loved ones, and being involved physically by taking walks, hiking, boating, kayaking, playing a sport, you will see a change.

Something to make you sweat and get the blood flowing will do wonders to your mind, body, and spirit.

Let's sum up this chapter with a quick checklist of how to avoid this "one thousand cuts" metaphor, and keep those bad habits and traits at bay.

Remember, one bad habit or "cut" a day may seem harmless, but over time they will be the most painful to have to bear. Let us change that.

1. Be willing to admit struggles in a humbling honorable manner.
2. Stop worrying about others, Be you, and focus on being the best you.
3. Be in fighter mode and be willing to fight for your values.
4. Write out a game plan on how to focus and maintain your values/dreams.
5. Doing things out of love is the answer when in doubt of your motives.
6. Be physically fit...the best version of you...no excuses.
7. Use positive ideas/tips to keep your mind sharp and clear of clutter.
8. Pray and/or mediate for clarity throughout the day as needed.
9. Whatever your daily line of work, keep positive, focus on your vision plan.
10. After a tough day at work, home and family are still needing you to be there for them. Use tips/ideas to walk in the door refreshed and ready for a positive evening.
11. Limit screen time/be in the moment more/have a positive evening routine/ set up and make sure to get 6-8 hours of sleep no matter what.
12. Repeat the similar plan the next day/adjust anything as needed to ensure that you are on the right path for you...keep some things routine and robotic, and make other things more adventurous and more in the moment. Just be the best you and enjoy your life. Good luck.

CHAPTER FIVE

BENNY

It has been a month after finishing the last chapter. This one has been tough to start. The fear of bringing pain back into my mind and soul is a challenging thing to convey. In the spirit of this book, however, bringing out darkness into light to live your best life, I need to share about how a small barking long haired chihuahua can teach you about life.

Social media has provided outlets for people to post their opinions, and facts on just about every debatable issue. Science books can now provide all the what, why, where, and how answers to the questions about life both on Earth and beyond. The Bible also contains the answers to how, why, what, and where questions about life after death.

While all of these methods of finding answers can be helpful and also truthful, in one way or the other, they only sound like the truth when your life is under control or you feel in control. I also thought I had many answers and control on life, that is until you don't.

When dark tragedy and raw moments happen, you and I will realize in a very real and raw way that we don't know anything, not a damn thing.

Those of you who still think you are sure of life and have control, none of us can fully attain it; it is a losing battle. You can fight the truth all you want, but surrendering to that truth will add such a calmness to your life. How many people do you know, including you and me, have used the words "always" and "never?" Those words are concrete in their saying. It gives a false sense of control over life. I can't even count how many times I have used those words and they have bit me in the butt when it does happen, or in the other case, doesn't.

I remember telling my family one of the ultimate "never" statements. It's a weird feeling to reflect back on a version of yourself. Depending on where you are in your life, you either look at it in disgust or maybe in some cases proud of yourself. In my case it was disgust.

I had always been a cat person since I was a child. I just disliked dogs for what seemed like lack of control of themselves. I would get uncomfortable going to other people's houses and have their dogs either barking, jumping, licking, or biting.

You could only imagine the look on my face when my family asked for a small dog. They tried to negotiate with me. I had said the ultimate statement years ago, "I will never have a dog in this house!" They knew it would be a tough sell, but they gave it all.

They had found this small chihuahua that needed a home. With all three of my kids being in that super cute innocent stage in their life and my beautiful wife who always wanted a puppy, I finally gave in. I figured it was so small that it could not be as bad as a bigger one, and with all of them around, I wouldn't have to do much with it. We picked up our first puppy named Lulu soon after that "negotiation."

She was a cute little thing. She didn't bark as much as I thought and, to my surprise, was a relatively calm chihuahua. She definitely won over my heart, and really changed my opinion about dogs.

I also started to have this feeling that because I softened my view on dogs, and noticed how Lulu would get excited to see other dogs that another question would soon pop up with my family. You guessed it, "Can we get another chihuahua so Lulu has someone to play with?"

I was more hesitant because two dogs would mean double everything. Double dog food bags, double vet bills, basically double trouble. I did notice that a companion for Lulu would be good for her, and since I had been won over a little by Lulu, that one more little one wouldn't be so bad.

Before I knew it, we were on our way to meet a little black long haired chihuahua. I knew as soon as we saw the cute little guy that he was coming home with us. He was in a crate and looked like he was in there a lot. We all felt the need to bring him home and show him lots of love. But there was one small problem. He didn't like me. He would bark, and try to bite me every time I would try to pet him, and take him from someone's hands.

He didn't want me in the same room with the family. He was a barker, too, well at least when I was around.

Then something crazy happened. We needed to go to the store, so my wife decided to take all the kids with her to see if maybe I could get some playing time with the new dogs and win their affection.

It worked. As soon as they walked out the door, I went and sat down on the floor of the living room and called to him. He instantly and calmly came over and sat in my lap like I had been his best friend all along. I guess I gave the first impression that I was a bad guy trying to hurt his new family, but now with them gone, and the time to think about it, we could now be friends. We named him Benny.

I felt like we added two new kids in the house. Benny and Lulu were running around with each other, and the kids were inseparable.

They both like to snuggle too. If anyone was on the couch or had a blanket, they were going to be there to be on it. We even took pictures and videos of them doing crazy stuff all the time.

Someone once said, "You need to ask yourself if you are an Eeyore or a Tigger living life?" Well, Lulu's personality was definitely an Eeyore being so mopey and basically wanting to lay around with someone on the couch with a blanket until dinner time, and then repeated the same behavior the next day.

Benny was Tigger times two. He still liked to be with people on the couch and snuggle, but he always ran around and checked up on what everyone was doing. He was very playful and happy all the time, too. He would leave his sock monkeys all over the yard getting into trouble. He made a lot of noise, too. He wasn't too crazy of a barker, but if someone was new in the house, it was full on crazy bark. He acted so tough, but really he was a lover, not a fighter.

We found out that he absolutely loved car rides. He was the perfect passenger. He was always good in the car. He loved looking around and seeing everything, which also made him tired. He would usually curl up in my lap for most of the car ride.

His hair grew crazy quick, so we had to get him doggy cuts often. He loved the car trips there, of course. We would drop him off, and loved picking him up, because he always looked very cute after.

He was such a protector for anyone in need, not that anyone was in life or death situations. If he noticed any of us play fighting, or we would sometimes pretend to be frightened, he would start barking at them to knock it off. It didn't matter if you were big or small starting it. He simply didn't like to see bullies.

To be transparent, his barking was the most annoying part about him. If someone came to visit, he would let you know you weren't invited. If he noticed anything different in the yard, or a neighbor next door, you might as well bring him back in because he would bark for 24 hours if you let him.

Just like other family members though, everyone has a couple little quirks about them, but overall they are great to be around. That is how I viewed him. I tried to push past the barking part knowing that dogs tend to do that, and he meant well by voicing his concern the only way he knew how.

A few years later we moved into a more wooded area lot. We started to have a harder time with them being out there hanging out. There were the new neighbors who would be outside from one of the fours sides of the yard, and that started the barking.

One of the neighbors had three big dogs, and we had a heck of a time keeping them away from that part of the fence. They always wanted to be over there checking it out, and barking 24/7 at them to tell them to keep away from us. Those dogs towered over ours, but you would have never known by their bark and aggressiveness toward them.

We finally had to build a giant cut off point for that whole part of the fence using our two sheds as a natural barrier, and then strategically placing five-foot tall stacks of firewood neatly between the sheds to block their view of the other yard and their dogs. Once in a while, you would hear their dogs bark, but other than all the dogs were out of sight/out of mind to each other.

Benny snagged his paw on the fence on Easter one day, and we had to make an emergency trip to the ER to stop the bleeding. Ticks were also heavy in the wooded area, so we constantly had to check. The biggest problem was the rabbits and squirrels everywhere. They loved to chase them, and they would give them a run for their money, even though I don't think they would know what to do if they actually did catch them.

Those creatures of the woods kept them occupied all the time, sniffing around the perimeter of the fence and tracking their scent. Over the years we became comfortable letting them out the sliding door. They would chase something, then go to the bathroom and usually we would call them back in after a few minutes, and they usually would come running back to us.

Life with our dogs was a true blessing to us. Here is something harsh about life, though. Things are always changing. Either for good or bad. Destiny or randomly happening. There are movements going on in the world that seem to have some kind of butterfly effect.

One of those things would be a bunny rabbit just looking for food in both our front yard and backyard, and needing a path to make that happen so it dug a small enough hole under the fence to squeeze through. The problem with that is quite a few small animals can squeeze through that same hole.

Including Benny.

I was just finishing up my day at work, and then headed to pick up the kids a little later after their practices. Then I received the most intense phone call I have ever experienced. There was a pause of someone trying to spit words out. The crying was so intense I couldn't understand what my wife was saying. After she repeated it, I barely understood the words that Benny was dead. There are moments in your life when time stands still. This was one of those moments.

I was overwhelmed with shock, but somehow I spit out the words "I'll be there as fast as I can. I quickly called my oldest daughter, and without telling her, told her to wait for practice to get out, and bring your brother and sister home later on.

I remember driving home fast and understanding that our life had changed dramatically from that moment on.

You see, an hour before Benny had been let out to pee and quickly found the rabbit hole entrance, he managed to crawl under and ran into the front yard and toward the street. Our street is not super busy, but life being what it is, a random car drove up our hilly road at the same time he ran out and hit Benny. The person in the car, knowing what happened, immediately drove away quickly.

My wife couldn't find him outside, and she ran inside and looked out the front window and saw Benny laying on the road.

I prayed as I drove. I knew I wasn't ready for what I was about to see. I prayed for strength, and also had this quote in my mind. "Don't mistake the presence of darkness for the absence of God." When I pulled into the drive, all that just seemed to disappear from my mind.

To this day, it was the most intense, emotional moment I have been through. I saw my shaking wife holding Benny in her arms sitting in the front yard. She was holding him like she always did, but this time there was no movement from him. I slammed the truck in park and ran up to her.

I cried the most uncontrollable tears I have ever shed. I literally lost strength in my legs and dropped to my knees and cried. I had this intense rage build in me. I thought I could handle life. It was like life stabbed me in the heart and slammed me to the ground. I remember hunched down on my knees, and with all the rage I had I yelled out at the top of my lungs "Fuck." I wanted to see Benny alive again, and that was never going to happen again and life just tore my heart out. I felt betrayed by life. I just turned to my wife and sat with her just crying and petting Benny.

We knew the kids would be home soon. We wanted the kids to remember Benny alive and not see him like that. We also wanted to give Benny a proper burial. The veterinarian offices were closed and yet we still wanted him to be close to us. We grabbed a tote and put all of his favorite blankets and favorite toys with him, and I dug the fastest and deepest hole I had ever dug. With literally blood, sweat, and tears we buried him in the backyard that afternoon.

A half hour later, the kids pulled in the driveway not knowing what happened at all. This painful day was not done yet. We sat the kids down and told them what happened. While they cried, we all did a family hug. We had lost a family member that day, and we knew life in our home would never be the same.

I wrote this two years later, and it's still very hard to reread it, and have the moment replay in my mind. To be truthful, it still often brings out anger and frustration most of the time in me about him being gone. I still have a hard time seeing cruel people getting away with things, and people complaining about stupid, unimportant things while Benny, who was sweet, kind, and innocent had to leave us. I know it is a weird way to think about the situation. I believe it was my helplessness about the situation that fuels that. My whole family is still very emotional about it, and I am right there with them. He was one of the reasons for writing another book.

They say time and the grief process heal deaths. Well, that's sugar coating it. It doesn't heal. It does move life forward in some ways, but here are a couple things I have learned dealing with death.

1. Time doesn't heal. It doesn't make it fade away either. Your memories will pop up when you least expect it. Something or someone says something that triggers a moment with them. They come and they go at random times. When they do, please try to put it in the back of your mind. Honor the moment and either laugh or cry with it. Acknowledge it, and hopefully move forward until the next moment arrives.

2. The grieving process is real, and those emotions are there. But for me they were not in an order like they are listed on many sites. I believe it depends on the intensity of the situation, but it goes like a roller coaster. Crying, smiling, anger, happy thoughts, frustration, blame, depression-like episodes. Embrace all of the emotions, and know life

unfortunately gives you these moments, and we must face the truth in front of us.
3. Death does one thing. It changes you for better or worse. Some people get even more sadness, angry, bitter, depressed, or even take their own life. Some people re-evaluate and re-prioritize what is important in their lives.

It was both for me. We dealt with multiple deaths that year. Each death made many of the above statements happen mentally to each situation. Benny's was more extreme because of the sudden, intense accident. Plus, we were extremely close to him, and the only one who lived with us for years.

Still, after a couple years, I have the same thought come over me and fuels my anger about life's unfairness. Benny was kind, and an example of what love is. In fact, many pets are. It doesn't matter your situation. Looks, addictions, struggle, personality. When you come home, your pet greets you with such love and affection for you. All they want to do is spend time with you, and be around you.

I remember seeing a bumper sticker one time. It read "Lord, let me be the person my pet thinks I am." I think of that often when I think of Benny's love for my family and me. It makes me smile, and press forward with life and try to live just like he did, full of love.

To have something so cruel happen to the innocent just tears me up inside. I am a person of faith, and it is (along with many others) still my biggest struggle. That is where my anger and bitterness remains.

I had never really become emotional watching movies or got emotional when I heard a sad story from someone or saw a sad scene in a movie. Since Benny's passing, every time an intense sad scene shows up in the movie, I would find myself getting emotional about it. If it involves a family losing a dog, forget about it, let the waterworks begin.

My family has seen me more emotional, and I am okay with that.
I want my family to see me, a strong man, showing compassion toward life's struggles, yet moving forward and learning more about myself. I don't need to hide my tears or emotions in fear of looking "soft" or less manly. My presence and how I handle sadness and compassion is the best way to show what a strong and kind man looks like.

As I mentioned above though, some moments are negative in thought, but other ways of thinking can become a positive for your life if you are willing to view life open-minded.

I read a powerful statement that has stuck in my mind for a couple years now. Frankly, it's a big part of what this book is about:

Everything starts with the truth. Nothing can be built without it!

This applies to everyone. As a man now, I'm speaking directly to all the men out there who are ready to seek the truth. I believe most men are not living this way. I know I wasn't. For me, coping with many deaths in one year opened my eyes to understand what type of man this world needs.

Men require reflection, being uncomfortable, and possessing courage that never ends. Being a man is a way of life, and it's made from everyday choices. We need to be more aware of our thought patterns.

We need to be strong, kind, and humble. Don't bully, whine, or judge. We need to stop blaming everything and everyone and create, and take responsibility for our lives. A true Alpha male is strong, smart, kind, calm, confident, and willing to help others. He doesn't need to boast. People will automatically know who you are by your actions. Words are cheap and don't mean much.

Confident men don't need to prove anything. Just focus on giving your value to the world instead of announcing it.

Simplify your life and you will start to find life in your life. Get curious about what is possible, accepting your story, start to make more uncomfortable decisions, and start sharing with the world your gifts, and the universe seems to have a way to make things move for you.

You may be wondering why I'm bringing those ideas to you now while writing this chapter. In honor of Benny, his death has transformed my self- centered little world, and made me understand that being a true man requires some of what I mentioned above. I needed to stop acting like a tough guy and think I have it all figured out.

I truly thought I was a man, while doing many things right in life. But in reality I had not even touched the surface.

Death does do one thing, it brings out the truth of what truly is important in your life, and what things really aren't that as important as you thought. No matter how much we try to hide from it, we must embrace it and let our true, inner emotions help us in how we live our lives moving forward from that point on, so that we truly can become over time the person our dogs think we are.

So here's a prayer I would like to impart about everything I have discussed.

God,

I'm still hurting badly. I'm angry at life, at cruel people, at allowed evilness in this world. I do have more empathy for certain people, and animals, but at the same time this unwanted anger of injustice and allowed cruelty frustrates me. I push forward and seek the light, but surrounded by darkness. I feel hopeless in finding the answers I seek. I have this logical and emotional battle in my head when trying to sort this world out. With pain in my heart, I carry on and want to fight the good fight. Protect me, carry me if you have to, but help me to the finish line, help show me the most honorable path I can know to get there, even though rough dark points occur.

CHAPTER SIX

CONNECTING THE DOTS

Do you remember in elementary school when the teacher would hand you a piece of paper with a bunch of random dots all over the paper, and by each dot was a number attached to it starting with one, two, three, etc? The instructions were for you to draw a straight line dot to dot in numerical order.

At the end of you connecting all the dots was supposed to emerge a picture of something. You can't visualize it at the beginning, because not enough lines are visible connecting the dots to form a mental image.

As you connected and formed a shape, that was when you were able to see ahead and know what would be showing at the end of connecting them. It was usually a cool feeling to see the image at the end, because your mind really couldn't place the image in your head at the beginning. But looking at it then looked cool because it didn't seem possible at the beginning.

When I was thinking of chapters to write about for this book, this parallel became something I believe to be relevant to finding your truth in your own life know matter what is currently going on.

Think of a piece of paper as your life. You have all these dots on there and they each represent a stage/area/choices in your life. So far, the dots have not formed a complete image. You have connected a few together but still no idea what the image is going to be.

The completed image will be the completion of your life, your life's work. It will take the effort of you connecting each dot together and letting each line connect together to start forming the image. It doesn't matter how fast you connect them. The most important part is connecting them to the right dots in the right way to form this image at the end.

This thought brings me back to my first book I wrote, "It's All About Faith, Family & Fitness." I had come to roadblocks in three main areas of my life. So, I wanted to show you how I was able to move forward and start connecting these dots in a more honorable way for myself, and what I cared about in and for my life. Hopefully you can relate to my thought process, and be able to use something in your life in those areas because many people want to move their life or "dots" in a more understanding way that fulfills them more in their life.

Starting with these three areas is a fantastic place to start. What I like about this connecting the dots analogy is that it takes away this whole start/finish quick completion of your life.

The dots represent not only years of your life but really the lines in between the dots which represent all of your daily choices/values throughout your life. The line in between the dots can cover so much life and the direction of it and how it will affect the completion of your image.

For instance, on the faith aspect of my connection of dots, my younger self had very little experience with it, and in my teens and early twenties I decided that faith was of no use to me.

I had a couple moments that happened early in my life that no matter all the evidence and logical thinking I had against faith, those remained as a solid reminder that no matter what I thought I knew it still was a mysterious thing.

One moment was during my childhood when we visited my Aunt and Uncle's church, which was different because we never went to church. I had visited with them before, and I had a good experience, but this time quite a few family members attended together. It was a Christmas Eve service. I remember it having this warm unique atmosphere.

There was positive music playing and inspiring messages being spoken. I remember them talking about a darkness in the world and how this light was going to save the world. I had no idea what the details of that were. I just had this feeling that everything was going to be OK, because this person they were talking about seemed so caring about us and had the power to do it.

I also remember back in high school after spending the day with my friends at the beach on Saturday. They said they had to leave to head back to school to be in the Baccalaureate ceremony, which is a spiritual event celebrating leaving high school and connecting faith to that experience.

I decided to go, since many of my friends were there, and I was intrigued when a good friend's father said a prayer while we were holding hands in a circle. I felt part of a family, and I felt this closeness to something I was unfamiliar with. To be a part of that with my close friends from school was an inspiring moment for me.

The most powerful moment and concrete evidence for faith in my life was the experience I talk about in my first book. During my favorite season, which was fall, I was on a field trip. I was walking alone from a gift shop to the pumpkin farm, and the weather was this perfect, serene autumn day.

Leaves were blowing around, the sky was overcast, and colors on the trees were in peak season. While walking and soaking in this beautiful setting, I suddenly had this overwhelming emotion inside me. It was the most beautiful "trance." I had this feeling of pure love, fulfillment, and gratitude. It only lasted for a few seconds, but to this day it was the most beautiful, raw moment that has happened with faith.

The reason for telling you those moments is not even trying to convince you to embrace faith or to provide some sort of evidence of it.

During all of those moments I knew nothing about faith or rebuked it. I'm telling you because I already know what nonbelievers think and feel about it.

I know we have strong animalistic behavior towards primates. I know how science has found answers for Earth and the universe. I know that the Bible seems to be this book of nonsense and magical thinking. I know how unfair suffering is in this world with God supposedly espousing to be this person of love. I know that disease and death are happening all over the world, and I understand there may be absolutely nothing that happens to us after death.

Here is what I feel is the truth. No matter how strong the evidence, there is still some level of uncertainty how faith and that mentioned above are connected. Those moments in my life were pure and unmotivated to find concrete evidence of faith. I wasn't even looking for them. The world didn't have influence and debatable arguments to persuade me. It was deeply personal and happened in silence.

I know you all have some moments in your life that only you know if they give some evidence of faith, even if you agree with the cases against faith. Deciding to involve faith in your life at some level is a stepping stone to how you will be connecting those dots in your life.

Oprah once said "some people make mistakes, some people call these failures. It's God's way of saying 'Hey, you are going in the wrong direction."

Take a look at the "dots" you have already connected in your life. Do the connections and the way life has worked out have some type of design or purpose look to it? Maybe you have more faith than you think you have, depending on how much life experience you have. The strength of your faith is directly related to your willingness to apply it to places you don't fully understand yet.

Even without fully understanding if faith plays a part of connecting your dots in life, embrace the pure, honorable parts of it, at least until you have more clear visions of it. Before connecting more dots in your life, stop and think about these thoughts.

1. When you start to think of goals, passions, and anything worthwhile in your life, what distractions usually pop up? Usually the more you start to act on those pursuits the more intense the distractions. That is resistance, or what I like to call darkness, and it's evil intentions. Resist distractions, and don't take the easy road, which is usually the common sense way to go. However, the soul will always seem to be uneasy and unfulfilled if you travel that path toward your next "dot." The answers are down the harder path to travel; it is designed to be that way.

2. Don't start your questions with "Will this make me enough money, or is this what others and society say I'm supposed to do?" Instead, ask "Will this bring more joy and wholeness to myself and others?" If you want to make yourself, your family, and others around you happier, get good at certain life skills, and your passions, and in return help others learn those who don't know it that will help their lives. It's such an emotional feeling to have someone come up to you later on and tell you because of you, their life has improved, and they have sincere gratitude about it.

I want to combine the last two main areas, because I feel you need to address these two more at the same time to see better results in your life—in the faith area that is more personal, which may or may not cause you to want to embrace your life; I respectfully understand that.

In your fitness journey and with your family, what changes need to occur, believe me, if you make even the smallest of changes, you will not be disappointed in yourself. You will feel proud and excited as you change them, and others will take notice.

No matter how many dots you have connected or what kind of crazy lines you have created while living your life, you can always correct your course and finish strong to get to the final image. You must be willing to understand and apply these ideas, though.

3. Acknowledge Failures and Successes. They are the same. They both help you move forward, and both can be huge motivation/wake up calls to take the step to change yourself.

4. Adjust your distractions. If it's an addiction/struggles, where you can get info/help to improve/eliminate? Is it too much time on technology or engaging in social media? What I have learned is we should be spending so much time investing and improving our own lives that we don't have any time criticizing others. Worry about you, and ditch excuses, because if it is important, you will find a way. If it's not, you will find an excuse.

5. One day at a time. It's easy to get overwhelmed thinking of all the changes you need to make. When you wake up each day, make a short list for each area you want to change, and also things that need to be done that day. Here is an example of a list I have made before in my life:

Do 10 push-ups today/1 mile run
Take five deep breaths at lunch to clear head
Take daughter to 3 pm dentist appointment
Organize bedroom today
Spend 15 minutes researching self help ideas
Take family out to dinner for some family time
Look over new way to pay down debt
Call mom/dad to just say hello

Now maybe half of those get done realistically at the end of the day, but you had a plan. And the list probably helped you get a couple more things done that you normally wouldn't have. Celebrate and acknowledge those "wins" you did that day, and before you know it your schedule starts aligning its way that you are improving in those areas at a fast pace. One day at a time.

6. Slow down and take action. Sounds contradicting, doesn't it? I just recently learned this and started to apply it to my life; it was a game changer. I was caught up in the hustle of life.

I was consistently staying busy, and being out of time with work, kids, family life, bills. I did some things OK, but most of my day was just getting by. I wasn't happy at work, and I didn't feel 100% committed/invested with my family. Bills were paid, but my wife and I wanted better results with our money.

I felt disconnected from friends and family. I saw others posting things on social media that showed them soaking up the good life.

Fortunately, I stumbled across a few videos from a couple Navy Seals, and one guy from the Christian influence. Even coming from different points of view, it was these two concepts: stop worrying about others' opinions, take control of your choices, eliminate distractions, simplify life immediately, and take a disciplined approach in every area that is important to you.

They also said you have to take action for all this to work. I wondered how you were supposed to slow life down, but also take action to start knocking the problems out of my life? I decided to give it a shot.

I deactivated from Facebook and Instagram accounts. I changed some things at work to make it more efficient for my family and myself mentally. We made a detailed plan on bills and budget and what we wanted for our future. I made fitness a top priority by getting a workout in every day and changed my nutrition intake with foods that gave me more energy, focus, and help with muscle growth.

I didn't worry about making social plans or what people were doing in their lives. I just went to work, came home and worked out, and spent more time with family at home. Social media was gone, which surprisingly made me mentally more at peace and more calm not having negative politics and news, debatable arguments, family drama, or keeping up with the Jones' negativity impact my mental health.

It was working. Focusing on myself and my family only really simplified my life; it gave me a new perspective on what I deemed important in my life. In a good way, I focused on and tried to be more disciplined in a few areas. It can do wonders when trying to start connecting the dots in your life:

-faith

-finances/ eliminating debt

-nutrition/working out

-very limited social media/technology

-quality family time

-work life more fulfilling

CHAPTER SEVEN

YOUR PAIN IS A PART OF YOU GREATNESS

As a huge Batman fan, I was excited that a recent teaser trailer was released of the upcoming film. It showed him walking slowly toward the camera in his famous bat suit. I noticed something different on the front of this suit that caught my eye, and I really wanted to talk about it in this chapter.

For those not familiar with the Batman story, his parents were murdered in front of him during his childhood, and that moment sparked what he stands for and fights for as a man.

In this trailer, I saw something I had never seen before. On the front of the suit were two pieces of a handgun taken apart, and put on the suit in a way that made it look like a bat. It's rumored to be the same gun that was used to kill his parents taken from the gunman himself.

Years ago I wouldn't have thought that much into it. Now, after dealing with pain and death since then, I embraced the idea. Some may believe that having such a constant reminder of that pain would make you full of rage, that you would consistently have the feeling of powerlessness where you can't control that pain, so you bury the guilt inside to avoid it. After all, the definition of pain is discomfort caused by mental suffering.

Sounds like a terrible way to live each day, until I learned about what could happen if you confront it and face the truth. Pain exists and always will be hovering over you daily, and must be fought back without hesitation, without pity for it. It will destroy you if you let it. The way to fight back is to reverse the pain and turn it into greatness.

I truly understand that statement is easier said than done. In fact, it's such a process that I'm still dealing with that method of changing my pain as I write this, but I know through some of the healing that I have gone through that it is the right direction to go to reach my full potential and the vision I have for myself.

The definition of greatness is standing out, all things working together at full capability and superiority. I'm not saying taking on pain and becoming great somehow makes you better than someone. It means that you are honoring your values and living a life of purpose that you should be and that the world could benefit from.

So let's dive into this idea. You see, the handguns on the bat suit aren't there for a reminder of the pain he went through. They are there to keep him focused and disregard imminent daily distractions, and harnessing that focus on real possibilities on using that pain for a drive that only emerges from emotions caused by pain. It is there to use that drive for changing yourself and the world.

First, a couple disclaimers. I know some pain is from very serious mental health problems, and I definitely recommend getting your doctor's advice on how to deal with your diagnosis before considering any information I discuss. I'm no professional, and I'm discussing my techniques and how I would and have dealt with some of these issues and emotions.

Second, I know some are dealing with pain that is physical, like loss of limb or having chronic pain from body injuries. I don't pretend to know your situation, or have answers to something I don't have some level of experience in. Please listen to all the professionals, and your own personal research and to help achieve what you want to do in the world.

The definition of greatness is widely considered to mean achieving perfection in something. We can all agree that life is far from that. I don't believe perfection is the end goal for our lives. The other definition of greatness caught my attention years ago, though. That is honor, living your purpose in life, all things working together at full potential.

Now, that is achievable. Easy to do? No. But just thinking about the possibilities I know is a path I want to at least travel down. We already know what happens to our potential in life if we don't travel that path...nothing.

When I learned about faith, and started to help kids through an after school program that helped change the direction of their lives, that was when I really realized how broken I was emotionally, and that I wanted to change years of bad moral and images of myself that I had consciously and subconsciously had of myself.

I first had to become self aware. I looked back and wrote down my past negative experiences, and I wrote next to them how I wanted to be more honorable and learn from them. I researched how to help change my mindset via online research, books, magazines, videos.

I surrounded myself with a more positive support group of family, friends, spiritual leaders, positive father figures, and people that were smarter than me in the areas I wanted improvement in. I still involved my fitness, and changed my nutrition, because I learned how important it was to keep my mental health in check, and how even the foods I ate affected mental health and emotions.

I didn't want my past to define me. I had to be careful, because I set high expectations for myself. At the same time, I had years of conditioned behavior and limitations for myself. I made mistakes and slip ups all the time, and became discouraged. Perseverance is a word to remember as you fall and get up, discovering a new you. Changes in your physical and mental health need humility and perseverance, as day by day you start to become who you want to be remembered for.

I researched the top ten negative emotions. and how to deal with them years ago. I want to share those emotions with you, and give you a personal experience of mine dealing with it. Remember, there is no conquering them; they are part of the journey as a human being. The emotions will come and go. It's a vicious cycle of beautiful emotions and dark emotions. I wish it wasn't, but life is what it is.

A few things I noticed before I told you these emotions. I have noticed many moments and experiences have combined emotions to them. You definitely get more than one at a time. I noticed that some people handle emotions better than others, and also how quickly emotions can come and go in any given day.

I can tell you that dealing with emotions and letting others see them is an uphill battle. First, I'm a man, and men are notorious for keeping emotions in and masking them. Second, I was raised by parents that have personality types that tend to keep emotion in more. Third, I also have a personality type that is very introverted, and emotions are one of the weaknesses of an INTJ type based on the Myer-Briggs personality test, which I highly recommend everyone do. But I will dive into that in later chapters.

The top 10 most common negative emotions are these:
Anger-Sadness-Fear-Guilt-Anxiety-Disappointment
Jealousy-Shame-Frustration-Apathy

Here are some examples of how this comes, and still is in my life at some level:

Anger, Sadness, Frustration, Anxiety--Dealing with the deaths of family and friends. Not having control of things I feel I am capable of handling myself. Seeing evil things happen in the world. Having goals and plans go up in flames because of life's chaos. Choosing to be less disciplined when I need to toughen up.

Anger, Anxiety, Disappointment
Jealously, Frustration, Apathy, Shame—Always looking at what everyone else has..always wanting more..questioning what people think of me..am I living up to their standards..my attitude toward others, my attitude toward myself..what's important and what's not to me living my life

Anger, Sadness, Guilt, Disappointment
Shame, Frustration—The mistakes I made as a husband, and father starting my marriage and raising my family,

missed opportunities in life, bad choices..bad attitude in life..when I know better and still screw up.

Sometimes your struggle isn't a result of what you're carrying but how you're carrying it. Wherever you are in life, take all the raw things in your life struggles, hardships put it all together to grow toward your vision.

I remember looking at my life's moments and starting to see patterns. I was making repetitive choices every day that usually had the same result. I would wake up everyday and wonder why things weren't changing. At that point I really wanted changes in my life, but nothing seemed to be changing.

Over time, it was really three things that really jump-started me into making small changes that turned into bigger ones later on at different stages.

One was that I noticed a repetitive pattern: I would wake up for the day and then soak in some motivation from some way and end up burning out by the end of the day. I'd tell myself that I must not truly feel or believe I want to become like that. Then I'd go to bed and repeat the next day.

What is the unofficial definition of insanity: doing the same thing over and over expecting the same result. Firstly, I found out that motivation is very short lived. It comes and goes often. Discipline was the answer for making those tough choices to keep moving forward long after the motivation fades away.

I also noticed my confidence was in the way. How can I learn new ways of thinking and developing new mindsets when my brain thinks it already has the answers from past experiences and knows more than most people.

Confidence is a good thing, but there's such a fine line that can take you over the edge quickly if you don't humble yourself often...and I do mean often.

Another trend I was seeing was how much I was looking into the past. I was daydreaming all the time trying to remember how things were so I could somehow get some answers. Unfortunately, I had so many bad qualities back then, making choices that my brain was just on repeat mode, and not humbling itself and thinking maybe I could try another way.

The mind will control you if you don't control it, and you need to understand how much control you actually have if you take it off cruise control and take over the wheel. It needs you to make humbling and tough decisions. Your mind can be childish, and you need to be an adult as much as possible.

The mind likes to be focused on either the past or the future thinking up schemes that usually are just dreamed up in the mind as it tries to act like it has all the answers. Focus on the present. The future will come soon enough, and it needs you to be focused and disciplined in the current moment making those choices, so your future will be better equipped by those choices.

I wanted to share a few breakthroughs that I had in my life, and how I have made some changes for the better in those areas. Firstly, I wanted to share the top 10 positive emotions, because they were extremely helpful in my journey of changing my life, and I know they will be helpful to others as well:

Joy-Gratitude-Serenity-Hope-Pride-Inspiration-Love-Awe-Interest-Forgiveness

I always wanted control of things around me. I always tried to keep a tight leash on things. I hardly shared my emotions to people, and I thought the whole world was out to get me. I had major trust issues.

I take ownership of that, though. No excuses. Some things I learned that have helped me dive into why that was, and still is at some level is a few things. I come from a family where every single person has gone through a divorce. I also have the personality type INTJ, which is very wired to be skeptical of things. Those two things combined are not good. I grew up seeing people leave each other all the time.

I saw people I trusted all around me give in to those raw human emotions when I thought they would come through.

I thought that I should be careful with my thoughts, because people at some point were going to betray me and take advantage of me, no matter how close the relationship.

I never had a strong foundation of those positive emotions mentioned above to offer advice on how to deal with divorce. It's always about changing and being accepting of new things and ways of life.

When I was looking at those ten positive emotions, and trying to find examples to write about something clicked with me at that moment. You need to be in the moment to be able to have those emotions. You usually need to be clear-headed and still not moving around, and just taking that moment in.

You need to not be in a hurry, or hustling, or trying to run a bunch of errands. You need just to be still. Take in the Joy. Acknowledge the Gratitude and Serenity. See the Inspiration and think about the Forgiveness of something/someone.

Trust me on this one, even to this very day as I write this. Slowing down and just reconnecting even for a few seconds is so necessary to living a more fulfilling life. I get so distracted by life about everything, but every time I humbly take a minute out of my "busy" day to just calm down, I never regret it. This happens to me multiple times every single day.

Seize the moments in your day and refocus your mindset by letting those positive emotions inside your mind to help you reconnect your thoughts and make better choices for you and your loved ones.

There is another extremely important idea we need to talk about, and that is speaking of taking a moment to adjust our thought pattern with emotions. This thought is one of the big steps of taking pain and using it for your greatness.

I remember listening to an interview, and the person said once he understood that success and failure were the same, it changed everything for him. It did for me too. I was always trying to avoid failure. Any day that I made screw ups or I disappointed someone, especially if they were close to me, I chalked it up to a bad day.

It took years to understand that success only comes after failure. Success requires being strong, kind, confident, humble, disciplined, and resilient.

I'll use my life examples to demonstrate this:

It took years of adjusting grueling workouts and trial and error on nutrition to get to a point of becoming strong and healthy.

It took learning from all the bad behavior, foul-mouth, negative thought patterns, and humbling my super ego to understand what I didn't want to come out of my mouth when talking to people. I started to become more self aware of how powerful worlds truly are. They are like weapons. They have power to lift people up or take them down.

Also the tone and sincerity of your words matter, I have also struggled with my tone and word use for years. Some people can have a calm nature about them when they speak, and it comes naturally. Some people like me have to work on how to soften your tone, and have a calming effect when speaking.

To my shame, I have a terrible history of using harsh tones and words. The consequences of your words and tone can be life changing. I almost lost my family because my demeanor was so degrading that my wife and kids would rather have me away, so the home environment would be more peaceful and not high strung when I'm around. Yes, I inherited this trait from a side of my family history, and my personality is wired to come off as sarcastic and arrogant. But I refused to use excuses to validate my history of offensive word use and tone.

I accept responsibility for my actions no matter how much I tried to make things change. We all need to take a step back for a minute. Think of how we truly want to live our life, and use our reflection, and research on ourselves to make better choices with our actions and image.

We can never change the past. All we can do is change the present and future by using the pain we experienced from the past, and make different choices based on what we learned from what not to repeat again in our life.

That probably is the most honorable thing we can do since we can't change the past. We can use it to help honor the present moments. That is the closest way to turn that negative past into a positive future.

Life is the ultimate teaching tool. From the start, the odds are against you from you living your life at your full potential. Through no fault of their own. The people raising us, parenting us, guiding us, mentoring us, probably has a mixture of positive and negative influence on us as we grow up. Life, both good and bad, has influenced them and so on and so on down the family tree.

For me, it has been a gradual process of flipping the switches on different aspects of my life, and all those trust issues I struggle with. I try to allow more positive people in my life, and rely and believe in them more,

In my younger years, I was not interested in school, and I goofed off. Now, I embrace education as a way to learn, and help show me new ways of living a better life for me, and how I want to lead my family.

I wanted to reflect on how I made bad choices and actions with my words and actions, and now I know how damaging that was, and now be more aware before I speak if I'm speaking out of negative emotions or positive emotions.

It sounds easy, but I know that it takes conscious effort to make changes.

Making small changes in your weak areas that usually cause pain at some level in your life will make a huge honorable shift in the direction of your life.

For me,
Trust more
Educate myself more
Overcome negative emotions more
Embrace positive emotions more
Discipline my finances more
Pursue my passions more
Reflect and adapt to life more
Exercise and eat healthier more
Love my family and friends more

Pain is Pain. There's no sugar coating it. What I have learned is to experience it, acknowledge it, and not forget it, but to use it as a way to appreciate life's precious time available. Honor the pain, but put action and choices into your life that you want seen at the end of your life as your greatness.

CHAPTER EIGHT

THERE IS A WAY

How many times do you believe people when they ask themselves, "Maybe life can be different today." I'm sure one of the millions of people who die of smoking-related deaths each year ask that question about them trying to quit smoking every time they try.

I know my aunt asked that question weeks before her death. I received the call from my mom that truthfully I knew would come sooner than later, because of her aggressive smoking habits.

My aunt had fallen ill, and was having trouble rebounding from it. I had a feeling that once blood work and x-rays were done, it would open the truth about years of smoking. Between my asthma and learning of second-hand smoking that I had been exposed to, I despised the addiction. It not only affected my health, but the people I cared about.

She was told that she wouldn't make it to the end of the year. I teared up as my mom told me the news. I also teared up as we walked into the hospital room to see her and talk to her. The truth was in front of us.

We both knew there was no fixing anything. She was going to be moved to the nursing home that my mom worked at, so she could also keep a closer eye on her while in this state. My aunt and I painfully knew she would not be leaving that nursing home.

Our whole family went to the nursing home to visit. Knowing time was limited, we enjoyed revisiting the past and laughing at good memories. The next time I visited her was the last time. I was told that most likely any day could be her last.

I seized the opportunity and made the most of the visit. Before I left her bedside, I wanted to ask her a question. I told her I was thinking of writing a second book. I asked her if there was anything she wanted me to tell people in the book that would help them out in their life? She thought about it for a minute. She was having trouble breathing and remembering because of the treatments and medicine.

She looked at me and said, "There is a way." She was referring to quitting smoking. There was a vision or a purpose in the way she said it. It wasn't in a voice that just said just quit smoking. It had a tone to it that said that it would be extremely hard, but it can be done. There is a way.

A few months earlier I ran into my aunt while I was working around town. It was the last time I would see her under normal circumstances. She told me she just finished reading my first book I just wrote. She mentioned she took heart to the part where I talk about addictions, and smoking was one of them.

She told me that it struck a chord with her, and she was going to quit smoking. To be transparent, she humorously was holding a cigarette while telling me this. I brushed the thought of her doing that, but I found out weeks later that she was telling me the truth. She did quit smoking, and when she was diagnosed with cancer, she hadn't been smoking at all. Smoking all those years was going to take her life, but not those last days of her life. Cancer won the battle, but she went out her way. Her final attempt of quitting was a successful one.

I found out that my book was an inspiration to her quitting, but the credit goes to her alone. She made the choice. Looking back on this moment, I now see the meaning of a few quotes I came across researching for this book.

Love is the reason for everything. Love is in everything, whether you like it or not.

You see, a pattern had to happen for me to be able to write about this now. My aunt's sin was smoking. We all have sin; it's just in different forms. We are all suffering from it, whether it is physical, mental, or spiritual.

In spiritual terms, sin is darkness, but darkness is not capable of overthrowing the light. It can't even comprehend the light. The light is Love, and if Love is the reason for everything, if you give that sin up, you will become a new person. That overcoming of darkness will now be used to show love to other people by using it as an example of how to overcome the so called indestructible sin.

She understood this in the end. It starts with you. You have to believe in yourself, and love yourself before you can even get started on helping others. She found her way.

So if sin lives in the darkness of us, that means it can't survive in the light of us. We need to bring it up from deep within us and bring to the surface to face it. One of the first truths to ask is are you fully committed? If you are not, stop wondering why you are not where you want to be until you decide to become fully committed.

A beautiful quote from the late Alan Rickman(Snape from Harry Potter) read, "I think there is some connection between absolute discipline and absolute freedom."

The way he used the words caught my attention especially when thinking of this chapter. One of the definitions of the word absolute is reaching a point that nothing is restricting it.

If your reasoning behind quitting, and your reasoning of the commitment of discipline is absolute, that means you have reached a breaking point in which no excuses can restrict you. You are beyond and above the excuses. The love you have for yourself has reached a level that the sin has never witnessed before, and can't comprehend it.

Once you reach that level of discipline, you will see the type of freedom that can only come from that level of love that you have for yourself and what you see yourself becoming.

Speaking of the word absolute, I believe we need to find the answer to this question if we really want to bring our dark addictions and struggles to the light. What is the Truth? Remember the word absolute means a level that nothing can influence. The Truth is the Truth. We can't sugar coat it, or white lie our way through it or around it.

So we start with the truth. Is this thing in my life slowly destroying me from the inside out? Just like the one thousand cuts analogy in the previous chapter, those small choices become bigger problems as life goes on.

Once you decide it's a problem, surround yourself with the resources and people needed to take it on. Get counseling if needed, surround yourself with only positive, and trusted people to counsel in.

All technology and social media should only be used for positive purposes. Unfollow and/or adjust settings so nothing that will be a possible distraction will slowly make its way to your screen.

Every morning, take a few minutes to visualize yourself making the right choices as your day goes that will be part of the plan to conquer this evil addiction and struggle.

Another point to mention, and it will sound selfish and emotionless to say, but you will need to give most of your attention to yourself to deal with this problem. What you are doing, though, is the exact opposite of what society will lead you to believe.

We can't fully love and lead our loved ones if we are not in a "growth mindset" frame of mind. There are two types of mindset, growth and fixed.
The fixed mindset is more of an "it is what it is", and "these are the cards I have been dealt." They believe that nothing is changing much, so they just complain each day about the problems.

The growth mindset sees opportunities to make changes to their situation whenever possible. They change and start taking charge of their lives in every area they have some control over.

Your loved ones need a growth mindset person in their lives for them to be able to grow and live at their best potential. They will have a difficult time doing that unless you invest the time and energy to take on your struggles. In return for the sacrificed time that you gave yourself instead of them they will be better off, as they move forward with their future lives.

Your short term intense concentration on your issues will have life changing effects on your inner circle of loved ones. Everyone at some point in their lives needs to make the tough decision on concentrating on themselves, and make life changing action steps, so in return your life and others lives will be better for it. It is not selfish; it's the opposite of it.

Every day in your life beyond the chaos that everyone deals with as the day goes on, always look for the truth and love in all that you do for yourself.

It's in the truth and the love that you will find a way.

CHAPTER NINE

A CHAMPIONSHIP TEAM

It's fitting that as I write this chapter, I'm watching "The Last Dance" documentary on the legendary Michael Jordan and the Chicago Bulls. It gives a glimpse on how the team was, and how and what happened for them to go after another championship. They were at the top of their game going for their sixth title.

I want to use their team as an example. I'm a huge Jordan fan. His work ethic on and off the court was extremely rare. He demanded full effort from everyone for each game and practice. To his credit, he never asked the team to do something that he already wasn't putting full effort into also.

He worked just as hard, even harder. That type of vision has a cost though. The rarity of that type of drive can easily be perceived as a negative way of treating people. Maybe there is a percentage of truth to that.

His response too was that he had the best intentions for that. To push everyone past their perceived potential, it was making them a better basketball player, and it helped them to win championships through that hard work. His intentions were honorable and was never intended to be like a villain to them. He was emotional talking about that topic, because it meant so much to him. But also he wanted his teammates to have the best experiences possible.

That style of leadership could still be questioned, but his teams did go to six championships all undefeated. Looking back, most teammates now see what he was doing, and they understood it now, and they talked about him with gratitude for that effort.

I want to share my sincere struggles, and also this drive similar to Jordan for how over the years having this vision of raising a family and having a sincere and long lasting marriage. We started as a young family, but our uniqueness individually and our unique way of visualizing a better future for us even from a tough start is what I believe helped us stand out and beat the odds.

It's foolish to say it is a total success story. There are many things I wish I could change. I want to share life hacks that we have learned along the way that could be helpful to others. It's about just trying to live an honorable life and be honorable mother and fathers.

There is no perfect family or a certain way to raise one. Raising a family is what life is. It can be fun, meaningful, purposeful, beautiful, gratifying, and humbling. It can also be tough, frustrating, draining, tiring, and resentful.

We can say the same thing about life, though, even though it is up and down with emotions and moments. It doesn't take away that at the end of the day, and in the moment you become "empty-nesters" All of those moments help define your greatness as a parent and spouse to them and yourself.

When building a winning team from scratch in sports, you need to have a plan or vision in place from the beginning. You know you are trying to get to a certain level of things coming together, but for a while you know things will be uncertain at best, setting up all the missing links and connecting the pieces.

As a young couple just married and raising a baby as teenagers, we had the odds and stats against us from the start. Marriage is a tricky situation from the start. You have two people bringing their goals, dreams, and talents together under one roof. Chaos, at least at some level, is going to happen. Here is the thing, though, if handled and done right it could become a beautiful thing.

I could have been such a better husband if only I had this advice years ago when we were arguing over different ideas and choices. Usually each other's goal is to show the other that they are right and the other is wrong.

Guess what? This isn't a competition. You are on the same team. The main goal for both people is to do everything to build up your family, not try to tear it down just to win an argument. Let me repeat this one. You are on the same team with the same end goal. Build your marriage and family, and move forward, not backwards.

On a lighter note, I once heard a singer say in an interview, "Keep the fights clean and the sex dirty." That is the case for us.

Showing that your marriage is a priority by your words and actions is another crucial element that needs to be part of your vision. Everyone at some point and level has a concern for oblivion in their life. The definition of that is basically the state of being forgotten. No one remembering you is a terrible place to end up.

In the movie "A Fault In Our Stars" a young man was dying of terminal cancer soon, and he never was going to make his mark on the world because of an early death.

His love interest asked of him, "Aren't I enough? I care about you deeply, and I will remember you."

I remember being ambitious and getting tunnel vision, trying to work my way to a point of being recognized as someone important, or even thinking I was needed to make this world better. Either by getting involved over the years with church programs, the after school program Five Star Life, different work positions, and writing and promoting my first book I wanted to be remembered.

Yes, some level of reaching out and helping the world is needed. But it's never at the cost of not having your marriage the top priority, though. Every time I start to aggressively spend time and energy and get off balance trying to help the community, my marriage and family suffered the effects.

Mother Teresa said it best, "If you want to change the world, go home and love your family." Change starts at home. Put full effort into your marriage and family, and they will see when you show strength, humility, forgiveness, and love. They will be inspired and changed by your leading example and go out into the world and lead by that example and inspire others to do it, too.

I have started to seek the truth in things as I become older. I was beginning to see how important my role was as a husband and father as time went on. The truth was I was capable of being a better man. I went into learning mode.

I believe the fastest way to become better is to put your ego in check early on. I'm not saying not be a confident man. You can't influence and inspire your family if you are not connected to them in some way.

I also wanted to spend more time with them, know how to communicate with them. I wanted to know when not to act on emotions and logic in certain situations. I needed to learn to be more focused and disciplined with my time, energy, and money. Basically, to put it bluntly, I had a lot of work and learning to do.

I wrote down my strengths and weaknesses and my visions. Confidence is knowing that you are very good at something, but you don't need to brag about it to everyone. Yes, I was strong and smart and had high energy and vision thinking skills, but more actual action was needed if I wanted to work on improving my weaknesses and low points.

I sought out anyone either online or that I knew who had my weaknesses as their strengths. I studied them or asked genuine questions on how to work on it over time.

I also learned that no matter what your strengths and weaknesses are, they can be useless, or even cause more problems if situations are at a certain point. What I mean by that is a struggling addict said he learned in rehab that there are basically four situations that if you find yourself in, you need to fix before you even continue with your day.

The situations can be summarized by using a keyword that conveniently means to stop everything: HALT

H stands for Hungry
A stands for Angry
L stands for Lonely
T stands for Tired

You have to admit, how many times when you felt any of those you have lashed out at someone, said something that maybe you normally wouldn't have said in a certain way. I truly believe we are, under those circumstances, a lot more often than we think.

Go eat some food, leave the room and calm down, call or talk to a close friend, take a nap or go to bed early. It seems so simple, but we fight those urges to better ourselves before reacting to something. Nine out of ten times we are talking to someone, because they are inside our life circle of people, and we need to be in the right state of mind, and not be in one of those four stages when around them. Humility goes a long way. If you are feeling not 100%, be truthful and tell them, and you will respond to them when you leave and take care of the problem.

So I learned that when I communicate that I need to remember that we are on the same team, and there is no reason to bring them down with hurtful or unnecessary tones or words that don't take your relationship to a more positive place. That helps nobody in the relationship.

I have also learned there are certain situations that should be avoided so when you do spend time together, you are feeling 100% and are in a positive and inspiring state of mind.

I took a free, 15-20 questionnaire personality test. There are two main ones used, Myers-Biggs and Enneagram. This changed everything about me. I didn't know that you can basically put people into 16 different types on how they are wired mentally. There were questions like if you are private or outgoing, logical or emotional thinking, and your take on the world basically.

What I found out about me is I'm an INTJ or a Type 5 on the Enneagram. I'm private, smart, logical, introverted, vision thinking, problem solving, high energy, knowledge seeking and not outwardly emotional.

I learned a lot of awesome positive traits but like any type there were lots of weaknesses, too, particularly with traits with communicating with my family. My lack of understanding with emotional thinking and needing alone space and my own time caused a great deal of tension.

I can't stress enough to take ten minutes of your day and take the free questionnaire online. It will give you the basic wiring, and understanding of your characteristics. You will be able to adjust and understand more about yourself and how you make decisions better.

It showed me ways to improve my weaknesses and understand people better, and I understood and could relate better with my family on how they saw me and how I saw them.

I looked up advice for my type, and it guided me to become such a better man for my family, but also for me personally. I became at peace with myself knowing I'm not alone, and there are people out there who think similar, and have helpful tips and shared struggles that I could relate better to now.

It led me to be able to find answers to many of the questions I had about pretty much everything I wanted to know how to better myself with.

If I had to tell you where to start to help yourself build a better life and better the "team", aka your family and close friends, I would start with these six categories.

I had extremely low points with everyone on the list and after seeking the truth on how to move forward, these will get you there the fastest. Create your championship team.

discipline/healthy habits

fitness/nutrition

your personality type

spiritualness

marriage/ relationships

finances/saving

CHAPTER TEN

STOP BEING AFRAID AND LET THE WORLD SEE YOU

This quote helped me years ago when I wanted to get more curious about my faith struggles. I had this passion and energy inside me, but I still had this idea that there was something holding me back. Finally exposing myself to the world through volunteering, I found out more about myself.

Everyone, including me has these insecurities we all deal with every day. We don't want people to take advantage of them or mock us. Social media even solidifies our theories on that. Yes, they will definitely do those things know matter what.

What I like about the title quote is that you can help the world, but it will be on your terms. Society, volunteer programs, and even churches tell you to just start volunteering right away because society needs help. What they don't ask or know is that maybe your schedule isn't ready for that. What they don't ask or know is you haven't figured yourself out or that you need time to recharge yourself.

Yes, we need to stop being afraid. That requires us to deal with our insecurities and struggles first. Give us time to figure out the best way to be in the world. The second part of that quote is let. You will determine how and when and how much you will give to the world. When others depend on you at home you don't want to sacrifice time spent away from them.

Once you feel comfortable with your self improvement you have been doing, you probably have a great way to spread your passion. If you are still undecided whenever you are excited about something, and it feels as natural as breathing when you do it, chances are that is your thing.

Finally, the last part is letting the world see you. As a private person myself, I can understand the instinct to keep to yourself. Look at the world now. You have politics and people trying to group you into certain stereotypes with everything you say and do. You have social media judging all your content that you post. You see people protesting and going to court over disagreements.

Yes, some people will just want to see the world burn. Heck, even from a biological standpoint human nature has strong tendencies. Even some of the personality types are not wired to naturally want to be helpful to others and be empathetic toward the world.

I know it sounds like a lost cause, but it is not. I have witnessed change from helping others, and it is life changing. Here is a more personal way of looking at it. Do it because it's not what they deserve, but what you believe.

Maya Angelo had a great quote, and I believe that once you truly know what you stand for and what your character is, it will be time to venture into the world.

"My wish for you is that you continue to be who and how you are, to astonish a mean world with your acts of kindness and continue to allow humor to lighten the burden of your tender heart."

That is so powerful. Look, you need to fight darkness your way. If you have a talent or passion, act on it. The world needs uniqueness and creativity. I understand the hesitation of exposing yourself to a cruel world, but people are craving leadership. We could show people by our actions and not just words that are not perfect, but we are sincere with our intentions.

People are clinging to anybody with ideas to change the status quo lately. I admit, some things don't need changed, but some things do need a new direction or a fresh idea. One thing that hasn't changed is the qualities that people admire in a leader.

In my opinion, most people who think they are a good leader just aren't.

Those men and women are a rare breed. That is why the world is in chaos, even though we have all these so-called great leaders. Here is a list of the most common characteristics of an admired leader. Do any people of power now have these? I sure hope so, but my guess is no, and we need to find ways and find people with these characteristics, and rise with them to make changes for the better.

Humility-Generosity-Confidence-Honesty-Gratitude-Understanding/Forgiveness-Courage-Passion-Positive-Creative-Empathetic-Self aware-Influencing-Open-minded.

I truly believe that most people, especially self-aware people who have been striving to be a better person processes many of these qualities already. You see, I know that because it takes those qualities to understand and want better lives for ourselves, and you can't obtain a positive life with negative behavior. You also aren't able to have a society that cares unless you have people in it that actually do care about it.

I believe in the idea that if first we get to know ourselves and choose the harder path of becoming someone that we are proud to be is the first step. Then allow that person to inspire our spouse, kids, friends, and inner circle.

The ripple effect really takes off from there when they show the world through those leadership qualities that you inspired them to take ownership of what and who they are responsible for. The butterfly effect is truly unstoppable when everyone's actions reflect true leadership characteristics, and they understand that strength is not optional.

I have so many family and friends who have helped me in more ways I can't list on a page. For privacy concerns I will not mention them by name publicly, but here are some public people that I have learned so much through their sharing of knowledge and experiences that they are willing to share.

These people have books, social media platforms, podcasts, blogs, and videos that have had a huge impact on my dealing with my life, especially the last three years.

Please support and embrace their knowledge to best help you on your own journey:

Jefferson Bethke

Joe Rogan

Jocko Willink

Tony Robbins

Ed Mylett

Jeff Cavaliere

Tim Ferris

Mel Robbins

David Goggins

Arnold Schwarzenegger

Jordan Peterson

Prince Ea

Tom Bayou

Lewis Howes

Dwayne Johnson

James Clear

Matt D Avalla

Aubrey Marcus

Gary Vee

Rich Roll

Clayton Jennings

If you are interested in taking the quick, free test online or on their apps:

-Myers Briggs personality test

-Enneagram personality test

**For further questions reach out to
jc79miah@gmail.com**

**If you enjoyed this book please consider my first book
also available on Amazon.com**

"It's all about Faith-Family-Fitness"
By Jeremiah Clark